Praise for
The Glucose Revolution and The Glucose
Revolution

"The concept of the glyc[...]
and bastardized by popular writers and diet gurus.
Here, at last, is a book that explains what we know
about the glycemic index and its importance in designing a diet for optimum health. Carbohydrates are not all
bad. Read the good news about pasta and even—believe
it or not—sugar!"

—ANDREW WEIL, M.D., University of Arizona College
of Medicine, author of *Spontaneous Healing* and *8
Weeks to Optimum Health*

"Forget *Sugar Busters*. Forget *The Zone*. If you want
the real scoop on how carbohydrates and sugar affect
your body, read this book by the world's leading
researchers on the subject. It's the authoritative, last
word on choosing foods to control your blood sugar."

—JEAN CARPER, best-selling author of *Miracle Cures,
Stop Aging Now!* and *Food—Your Miracle Medicine*

"Although the jury is still out on the utility of the
glycemic index, many of the curious will benefit from a
careful reading of this book, and some will find that the
glycemic index is particularly helpful for them. Everyone
can enjoy the recipes, some of which are to die for!"

—JOHANNA DWYER, D. Sc., R.D., Editor,
Nutrition Today

OTHER *GLUCOSE REVOLUTION* TITLES

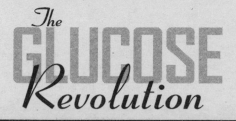

The GLUCOSE Revolution

POCKET GUIDE TO

LOSING WEIGHT

KAYE FOSTER-POWELL, M. NUTR. & DIET.
JENNIE BRAND-MILLER, PH.D.
THOMAS M.S. WOLEVER, M.D., PH.D.
STEPHEN COLAGIURI, M.D.

ADAPTED BY
JOHANNA BURANI, M.S., R.D., C.D.E.
AND LINDA RAO, M.ED.

■

MARLOWE & COMPANY
NEW YORK

Published by
Marlowe & Company
841 Broadway, 4th Floor
New York, NY 10003

This book is not intended to replace the services of a physician or dietitian. Any application of the recommendations set forth in the following pages is at the reader's discretion. The reader should consult with his or her own physician or dietitian concerning the recommendations in this book.

Copyright © text 1998, 2000 Kaye Foster-Powell, Jennie Brand-Miller, Thomas M.S. Wolever, Stephen Colagiuri

First published in Australia in 1998 in somewhat different form under the title *Pocket Guide to the G.I. Factor and Losing Weight* by Hodder Headline Australia Pty Limited.

This edition is published by arrangement with Hodder Headline Australia Pty Limited.

Library of Congress Cataloging-in-Publication Data
Brand-Miller, Janette, 1952-
     [Pocket guide to the G.I. factor and losing weight]
     The glucose revolution pocket guide to losing weight / by
Jennie Brand-Miller, Stephen Colagiuri [sic], Kaye Foster-Powell.
     p. cm.
     Australian text published in 1998 under the title: The pocket guide to the G.I. factor and losing weight.
     ISBN 1-56924-677-7
     1. Reducing diets—Handbooks, manuals, etc.   2. Glycemic index—Handbooks, manuals, etc.   I. Colagiuri, Stephen.   II. Foster-Powell, Kaye.   III. Title.

RC222.2.B66 2000
613.2'5—dc21
                                                                99-042189

9 8 7 6 5
Designed by Pauline Neuwirth, Neuwirth & Associates, Inc.
Distributed by Publishers Group West
Manufactured in the United States of America

CONTENTS

PREFACE

The Glucose Revolution is the definitive, all-in-one guide to the glycemic index. Now we have written this pocket guide to show you how the glycemic index (G.I.) can help you to lose weight. We know that low G.I. Foods have two very special advantages for people who want to lose weight:

- they fill you up and keep you satisfied for longer;
- they help you burn more of your body fat and less of your stored carbohydrate.

This book offers more in-depth information about using the glycemic index to lose weight than we had room to include in *The Glucose Revolution*. Much new information appears in this book that is not in *The Glucose Revolution*, including the questions most frequently asked by dieters about the glycemic index, a week's worth of low-G.I. meal plans, and success stories about people who have lost weight by making the switch to low-G.I. foods.

This book has been written to be read alongside *The Glucose Revolution*, so in the event you haven't already consulted that book, please be sure to do so, for a more comprehensive discussion of the glycemic index and all its uses.

Chapter 1

YOU NEED THIS BOOK

WHY DIETS DON'T WORK

QUANTITY ISN'T THE ISSUE—
THE GLYCEMIC INDEX IS

*Y*ou can't go anywhere these days without people talking about what they're eating—and *not* eating. It seems everyone's uttering those five golden words: "I'm on a new diet." But would you believe that even with all those diets, the number of overweight and obese people in our society is actually *climbing*? In fact, during the 1990s alone, the number of adult Americans has grown by what some experts are calling "epidemic" proportions: almost 50 percent! (The number of obese people in the state of Georgia, for example, has grown more than 100 percent over the past decade.)

The problem is so pervasive that some studies find 55 percent of American adults weighing more than they should. Worse yet, if this trend continues, experts say that within just a few generations, *every adult American* will be overweight! And excess weight brings with it a host of other health problems too, such as heart disease, diabetes, some types of cancer and high blood pressure.

NO LAUGHING MATTER

One study, conducted at St. Luke's/Roosevelt Medical Center in New York City, found that 325,000 deaths in the U.S. each year can be attributed to obesity. That makes obesity the *second leading cause of preventable death*—surpassed only by smoking.

America's weight problem isn't surprising, you may think, given the abundance of foods available to us. We eat away from home more often than we used to and consume greater amounts of fast and snack foods than ever before. As a nation, we were doing better for a while, when reported intakes of fat and calories were going down, but new research shows that the trend for fat consumption is now drifting back up.

WHY DIETS DON'T WORK

If you are overweight (or consider yourself to be) chances are that you have looked at countless books, brochures and magazines offering a solution to losing weight. New diets or miracle weight-loss solutions seem to appear weekly. They are clearly good for selling magazines, but for the majority of people who are overweight "diets" just don't work. If they did, there wouldn't be so many!

At best, a diet will reduce your calorie intake. At worst, it will change your body composition for the fatter. The reason? Many diets teach you to reduce your carbohydrate intake to bring about quick weight loss. The weight you lose, however, is mostly water (that was trapped or held with stored carbohydrate) and eventually muscle (as it is broken down to produce glucose). Once you return to your former way of eating, you regain a little bit more fat. With each desperate repetition of a diet, you lose more muscle. Over a course of years, the resultant change in body composition to less muscle and more fat makes it increasingly difficult to lose weight.

■

FOR THE MAJORITY OF PEOPLE WHO ARE OVERWEIGHT,
MAGAZINE "MIRACLE DIETS" DON'T WORK.
IF THEY DID, THERE WOULDN'T BE SO MANY OF THEM.

■

QUANTITY ISN'T THE ISSUE—
THE GLYCEMIC INDEX IS

When it comes to losing weight, it's not simply a matter of reducing how much you eat. Research (in Australia and other countries) has shown that the type of food you give your body determines which fuel it's going to burn and which it's going to store as body fat. Studies have also revealed that certain foods are much more satisfying than others. This is where the glycemic index (G.I.) comes into the picture: The glycemic index of foods is simply a ranking of foods based on their immediate effect on blood sugar levels. Carbohydrate foods that break down quickly during digestion have the highest G.I. values, and their blood sugar response is fast and high. Carbohydrates that break down slowly, releasing glucose gradually into the blood stream, have a low glycemic index.

Low G.I. foods have two very special advantages for people who want to lose weight: They fill you up and keep you satisfied for longer and they help you burn more of your body fat and less of your body muscle.

If you're trying to lose weight, low G.I. foods will enable you to increase your food intake without increasing your waistline, control your appetite and choose the right carbohydrates for your lifestyle and your well-being.

Indeed, good news lies in the pages ahead, because we're bringing you the very latest information about how low G.I. foods can help you lose weight and keep it off—for good. We offer you:

- scientific evidence about controlling your body weight;
- details about how the glycemic index can be used to best support your weight loss efforts;
- tips on how to put the glycemic index into practice;
- practical hints for changing your eating habits;
- a week of low G.I., low calorie menus plus a nutritional analysis for each menu and its glycemic index; and
- an A–Z listing of over 300 foods with their G.I., carbohydrate and fat content.

THERE'S NO NEED TO FEEL HUNGRY
WHEN YOU'RE LOSING WEIGHT

When you use the glycemic index (G.I.) as the basis for your food choices, you **DON'T** need to overly restrict your food intake, obsessively count calories or starve yourself.

Chapter 2

THE GLYCEMIC INDEX: SOME BACKGROUND

WHAT IS THE GLYCEMIC INDEX?

The glycemic index of foods is simply a ranking of foods based on their immediate effect on blood sugar levels. To make a fair comparison, all foods are compared with a reference food such as pure glucose and are tested in equivalent carbohydrate amounts.

Originally, research into the glycemic index of foods was inspired by the desire to identify the best foods for people with diabetes. But scientists are now discovering that G.I. values have implications for everyone.

Today we know the glycemic index of hundreds of different food items—both generic and name brand—that have been tested following a standardized testing method. The tables in Chapter 18 on pages 96 to 108 give the glycemic index of a range of common foods, including many tested at the University of Toronto and the University of Sydney.

THE GLYCEMIC INDEX MADE SIMPLE

Carbohydrate foods that break down quickly during digestion have the highest G.I. values. The blood glucose, or sugar, response is fast and high. In other words the glucose in the bloodstream increases rapidly. Conversely, carbohydrates that break down slowly, releasing glucose gradually into the bloodstream, have low G.I. values. An analogy might be the popular fable of the tortoise and the hare. The hare, just like high G.I. foods, speeds away full steam ahead but loses the race to the tortoise with his slow and steady pace. Similarly, slow and steady low G.I. foods produce a smooth blood sugar curve without wild fluctuations.

For most people most of the time, the foods with low G.I. values have advantages over those with high G.I. values. Figure 1 shows the effect of slow and fast carbohydrate digestion on blood sugar levels.

The substance that produces the greatest rise in blood sugar levels is pure glucose itself. All other foods have less effect when fed in equal amounts of carbohydrate. The glycemic index of pure glucose is set at 100, and every other food is ranked on a scale from 0 to 100 according to its actual effect on blood sugar levels.

The glycemic index of a food cannot be predicted from its composition or the glycemic index of related foods. To test the glycemic index, you need real people

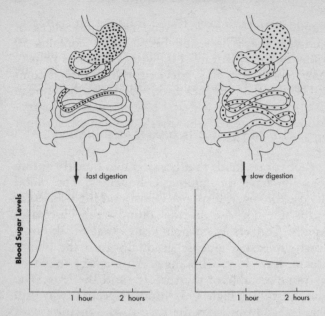

Figure 1. Slow and fast carbohydrate digestion and the consequent levels of sugar in the blood.

and real foods. We describe how the glycemic index of a food is measured in the following section. There is no easy, inexpensive substitute test. Scientists always follow standardized methods so that results from one group of people can be directly compared with those of another group.

In total, 8 to 10 people need to be tested and the glycemic index of the food is the average value of the group. We know this average figure is reproducible and that a different group of volunteers will produce a similar result. Results obtained in a group of people with diabetes are comparable to those without diabetes.

The most important point to note is that all foods are tested in equivalent carbohydrate amounts. For example, 100 grams of bread (about 3½ slices of sandwich bread) is tested because this contains 50 grams of carbohydrate. Likewise, 60 grams of jelly beans (containing 50 grams of carbohydrate) is compared with the reference food. We know how much carbohydrate is in a food by consulting food composition tables, the manufacturer's data or measuring it ourselves in the laboratory.

■

THE GLYCEMIC INDEX IS A CLINICALLY PROVEN TOOL IN ITS APPLICATIONS TO DIABETES, APPETITE CONTROL AND REDUCING THE RISK OF HEART DISEASE.

■

MEASURING THE GLYCEMIC INDEX

Scientists use just six steps to determine the glycemic index of a food. Simple as this may sound, it's actually quite a time-consuming process. Here's how it works.

1. An amount of food containing 50 grams of carbohydrate is given to a volunteer to eat. For example, to test boiled spaghetti, the volunteer would be given 200 grams of spaghetti, which supplies 50 grams of carbohydrate (we work this out from food composition tables or by measuring the available carbohydrate)—50 grams of carbohydrate is equivalent to 3 tablespoons of pure glucose powder.

2. Over the next two hours (or three hours if the volunteer has diabetes), we take a sample of their blood every 15 minutes during the first hour and thereafter every 30 minutes. The blood sugar level of

these blood samples is measured in the laboratory and recorded.

3. The blood sugar level is plotted on a graph and the area under the curve is calculated using a computer program (Figure 2).

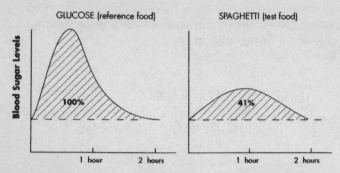

Figure 2. Measuring the glycemic index of a food. The effect of a food on blood sugar levels is calculated using the area under the curve (shaded area). The area under the curve after consumption of the test food is compared with the same area after the reference food (usually 50 grams of pure glucose or a 50 gram carbohydrate portion of white bread).

4. The volunteer's response to spaghetti (or whatever food is being tested) is compared with his or her blood sugar response to 50 grams of pure glucose (the reference food).

5. The reference food is tested on two or three separate occasions and an average value is calculated. This is done to reduce the effect of day-to-day variation in blood sugar responses.

6. The average glycemic index found in 8 to 10 people is the glycemic index of that food.

5 KEY FACTORS THAT INFLUENCE THE GLYCEMIC INDEX

Cooking methods

Cooking and processing increases the glycemic index of a food because it increases the amount of gelatinized starch in the food. Cornflakes is one example.

Physical form of the food

An intact fibrous coat, such as that on grains and legumes, acts as a physical barrier and slows down digestion, lowering a food's G.I. value.

Type of starch

There are two types of starch in foods, amylose and amylopectin. The more amylose starch a food contains, the lower the glycemic index.

Fiber

Viscous, soluble fibers, such as those found in rolled oats and apples, slow down digestion and lower a food's glycemic index.

Sugar

The presence of sugar, as well as the type of sugar, will influence a food's glycemic index. Fruits with a low glycemic index, such as apples and oranges, are high in fructose.

Chapter 3

FIXING A "BROKEN" DIET

WITH A WAVE OF THE FAT WAND . . .

WHAT'S WRONG WITH OUR WAY OF EATING?

WHY WE NEED TO EAT MORE CARBOHYDRATE

WHAT IS A BALANCED DIET?

Today's Western diet is the product of industrialization based on inventions ranging from Jethro Tull's seed drill (in 1701) to the high speed steel roller mills for milling cereals (in the nineteenth century) and advances in processing food to give it a longer shelf life. The benefits are many: We have plenty of relatively cheap, palatable (some would say too palatable) and safe foods available, and gone are the days of monotonous fare, gaps in the food supply and weevil-infested and adulterated food. Also long gone are widespread vitamin deficiencies such as scurvy and pellagra. Today's food manufacturers work hard to bring us irresistible products that meet the demands of both gourmets and health conscious consumers.

Many of the new foods are still based on our staple cereals—wheat, corn, and oats—but the original grain has been ground down to produce fine flours that yield the best quality breads, cakes, cookies, breakfast cereals and snack foods.

Cereal chemists and bakers know that the finest particle size flour produces the most palatable and shelf-stable end products. But this striving for excellence in one area has resulted in unforeseen problems in another. Today's staple carbohydrate foods, including some ordinary breads, are quickly digested and absorbed, and the resulting effect on blood sugar levels has created a problem for many of us.

■

TRADITIONAL DIETS ALL AROUND THE WORLD CONTAINED SLOWLY DIGESTED AND ABSORBED CARBOHYDRATE—FOODS WITH A LOW GLYCEMIC INDEX. IN CONTRAST, MODERN DIETS WITH THEIR QUICKLY DIGESTED FINE WHITE FLOURS ARE BASED ON FOODS WITH A HIGH GLYCEMIC INDEX.

■

WITH A WAVE OF THE FAT WAND . . .

The other undesirable aspect of the modern diet is its high fat content. Food manufacturers, bakers and chefs know we love to eat fat. We love its creaminess and mouth feel and find it easy to consume in excess. It makes our meat more tender, our vegetables and salads more palatable and our sweet foods even tastier. We prefer potatoes as French fries or potato chips, to have our fish battered and fried, and our pastas in rich creamy sauces. With a wave of the fat wand, bland high carbohydrate foods such as rice and oats are magically transformed into delicious, calorie-laden foods such as fried rice and sweetened granola. In fact, when you analyze it, much of our dict today is an unwanted but delicious combination of both fat and quickly digested carbohydrate.

WHAT'S WRONG WITH OUR WAY OF EATING?

- The modern diet is too high in saturated fat and too high in quick-release carbohydrate.
- The carbohydrate we eat is digested and absorbed too quickly because most modern starchy foods have a high glycemic index.

WHY WE NEED TO EAT MORE CARBOHYDRATE

For once, health experts are nearly unanimous. Most agree that the food we eat for breakfast, lunch and dinner and for those in-between snacks should be low in fat and high in carbohydrate. The same diet that helps prevent our becoming overweight also reduces our risk of developing heart disease, diabetes and many types of cancer.

But the story doesn't end there. To reduce the fat content of our diet, we need to eat more carbohydrate. In fact, carbohydrate should be the main source of calories in our food—not fat. Carbohydrate and fat have a reciprocal relationship in our diets: If we eat more high carbohydrate foods, they tend to displace the high fat foods from our diet. The new emphasis on eating lots of high carbohydrate foods has focused attention on the differences among carbohydrates.

WHAT IS A BALANCED DIET?

It makes sense to balance our food intake with the rate our bodies use it in order to maintain a steady weight. These days, however, this balance is difficult to achieve, since it's so easy to overeat. Refined foods, convenience foods and fast foods frequently lack fiber and conceal fat so that before we feel full, we have overdosed on calories. It is even easier not to exercise. It takes longer to walk somewhere than it does to drive (except perhaps in rush hour). With intake exceeding output on a regular basis, the result for too many of us is gaining weight.

We need to adapt our lifestyle to our high caloric diet and fewer physical demands. It's become very important to catch bursts of physical activity wherever we can to increase our energy output. (See Chapter 7 on page 38 for more information on exercise.)

While you work on increasing your energy output, the glycemic index can help you select the best foods to balance your intake. Its high carbohydrate basis ensures a filling diet that isn't packed with calories.

Chapter 4

LOSE WEIGHT
THE LOW G.I. WAY

WHY "FATTENING"
DOESN'T MEAN "FILLING"

EAT MORE, WEIGH LESS

DO YOU HAVE A WEIGHT PROBLEM?

A HEALTHY WEIGHT DISTRIBUTION

IS YOUR WEIGHT AFFECTING
YOUR HEALTH AND EVERYDAY LIFE?

WHAT WE REALLY NEED TO EAT
FOR HEALTH AND GROWTH

CUT THE FAT

*O*ne of the toughest aspects of trying to lose weight can be feeling hungry all the time. But a gnawing, empty feeling isn't necessary when you're shedding excess pounds. In fact, carbohydrates are natural appetite suppressants, because gram for gram, those carbohydrate foods with a low glycemic index are the most filling and prevent hunger pangs for longer periods of time.

In the past, experts believed that protein, fat and carbohydrate foods, taken in equal quantities, satisfied our appetites equally. We now know from recent research that the satiating (making us feel full) capacity of these three nutrients is *not* equal.

■ ■ ■

WHY "FATTENING" DOESN'T MEAN "FILLING"

Fatty foods have only a weak effect on satisfying appetite relative to the number of calories they provide. In an experimental situation, volunteers will consistently overconsume calories if they are offered foods that are high in fat. When high carbohydrate and low fat foods are offered, they consume fewer calories, eating to satisfaction, not fullness. That's why carbohydrate foods are the best for satisfying your appetite without oversatisfying your caloric requirement.

■

YOU CAN EAT QUANTITY—JUST CONSIDER THE QUALITY!

■

In studies conducted at the University of Sydney, people were given a range of individual foods that contained equal numbers of calories, then the satiety (feeling of fullness and satisfaction after eating) responses were compared. The researchers found that the most filling foods (such as potatoes, oatmeal, apples, oranges and pasta) were high in carbohydrate, which contains fewer calories per gram than other nutrients. Eating more of these foods satisfied appetite without providing excess calories. On the other hand, high fat foods, which provide many calories per gram, such as croissants, chocolate and peanuts, were the least satisfying. These foods help you store more fat and are less filling to eat. Low G.I. foods are even more filling than high G.I. foods. In fact, the lower the glycemic index, the fuller you'll feel.

Many people notice that eating extra carbohydrate at a meal tends to be compensated by eating less food at the next meal. When we eat more carbohydrate, the body responds by increasing its production of glycogen. Glycogen is stored as glucose, the critical fuel for our brain and muscles. The size of these stores is limited, however, and they must be continuously refilled by carbohydrate from the diet. Good glycogen stores ensure a well fueled body and make it easier to exercise. Even when we're not exercising, the body will use carbohydrate in preference to other fuel sources, because it is attempting to match the source of calories to the type of calories used.

■

EATING TO LOSE WEIGHT WITH LOW G.I. FOODS
IS EASIER BECAUSE YOU DON'T HAVE TO GO HUNGRY
AND WHAT YOU END UP WITH IS TRUE FAT LOSS.

■

By eating a high carbohydrate diet you will tend to automatically lower your fat intake, and by choosing your carbohydrate from low G.I. foods, you make meals and snacks even more satisfying.

THE PANCREAS PRODUCES INSULIN

The pancreas is a vital organ near the stomach, and its main job is to produce the hormone insulin. Carbohydrate stimulates the secretion of insulin more than any other component of food. The slow absorption of the carbohydrate in our food means that the pancreas doesn't have to work so hard and needs to produce less insulin. If the pancreas is overstimulated over a long period of time, it may become "exhausted" and type 2 diabetes can develop in genetically susceptible people. Even without diabetes, high insulin levels are undesirable because they increase the risk of heart disease.

Unfortunately, over time, we have begun to eat more "refined" foods and fewer "whole" foods. This new way of eating has brought with it higher bood sugar levels after a meal and higher insulin responses, as well. Though our bodies do need insulin for carbohydrate metabolism, high levels of the hormone have a profound effect on the development of many diseases. In fact, medical experts now believe that high insulin levels are one of the key factors responsible for heart disease and hypertension. Insulin influences the way we metabolize foods, determining whether we burn fat or carbodhydrate to meet our energy needs and ultimately determining whether we store fat in our bodies.

EAT MORE, WEIGH LESS

Even when the caloric intake is the same, people eating low G.I. foods may lose more weight than those eating high G.I. foods. In a study in South Africa, the investigators divided overweight women into two groups: One group ate a low calorie, high G.I. diet and the other, a low calorie, low G.I. diet. The amount of calories, fat, protein, carbohydrate and fiber in the diet was the same for both groups—only the glycemic index of the diets was different. The low G.I. group included foods such as lentils, pasta, oatmeal and corn in their diet and excluded high G.I. foods, including white bread. After 12 weeks, the volunteers in the group eating low G.I. foods had lost, on average, 20 pounds—4½ pounds more than people in the group eating the diet of high G.I. foods.

The most significant finding? The two diets affected blood levels of insulin completely differently. Low G.I. foods resulted in lower levels of insulin circulating in the bloodstream. Insulin, you'll remember, is a hormone that is not only involved in regulating blood sugar levels, but also plays a key part in when and how we store fat. High levels of insulin often exist in obese people, in those with high blood fat levels (either cholesterol or triglyceride) and those with heart disease. This study suggested that the low insulin responses associated with low G.I. foods helped the body to burn more fat rather than store it.

■

THE REAL AIM IN LOSING WEIGHT IS LOSING BODY FAT. PERHAPS IT WOULD BE BETTER DESCRIBED AS "RELEASING" BODY FAT. AFTER ALL, TO LOSE SOMETHING SUGGESTS THAT YOU HOPE TO FIND IT AGAIN SOME DAY!

■

If you are still fearful of gaining weight by eating more pasta, bread and potatoes, consider this: The body actually has to use up calories to convert the carbohydrate we eat into body fat. The cost is 23 percent of the available calories—that is, nearly one-quarter of the calories of the carbohydrate are used up just storing it. Naturally, the body is not inclined to waste energy this way. In fact, the body converts carbohydrate to fat only under very unusual situations such as forced overfeeding. The human body prefers the easy option, which is to burn those calories, and it is far more willing to add to our fat stores with the fat that we eat. Conversion of fat in food to body fat is an extremely efficient process and body fat stores are virtually limitless.

DO YOU HAVE A WEIGHT PROBLEM?

In putting together a book for weight loss we are only too well aware of the pressure many people feel to lose weight. We don't intend to add to that pressure. In fact, we suggest you clarify in your own mind whether your weight really is a problem to you.

It's worth doing an assessment of your situation to clarify your goals as far as your body weight is concerned. Here are some questions you need to ask yourself:

- Do you feel too fat?
- Is your weight contributing to poor health?
- Is your weight impacting on your daily life?
- Do you really want to lose weight?
- Why are you overweight?

■

ARE YOU AN APPLE OR A PEAR?
YOUR WAIST CIRCUMFERENCE SHOULD BE LESS THAN 35
INCHES (WOMEN) OR LESS THAN 39 INCHES (MEN).

■

A HEALTHY WEIGHT DISTRIBUTION

A weight-for-height chart can show you a range of weights that is considered healthiest for your height, but these charts aren't appropriate for everyone.

People from different populations around the world can't always be compared on the same scale. Some people tend to be smaller (lighter and shorter), while others, on the other hand, appear heavy in proportion to their height because of their muscle bulk. This doesn't mean they are unhealthy. A large mass of body fat on the other hand, is associated with health risk. This is true especially when the fat is centrally located—around the middle of your body in the waist, stomach and abdomen—which gives some people an "apple" shape. Women often carry a lot of fat on their hips, thighs and buttocks, giving them a "pear" shape. (This lower body fat is an energy store for reproduction and carries little health risk.) You can tell if you have too much fat around your middle by measuring your waist with a tape measure. Keep in mind that a waist circumference greater than 35 inches (females) or 39 inches (males) is too big.

CONSIDER THIS

If you eat healthy foods most of the time and do some type of physical activity for at least 30 minutes 4 to 5 times a week, then your size and shape may be right for you.

IS YOUR WEIGHT AFFECTING YOUR HEALTH AND EVERYDAY LIFE?

Unfortunately, if you are overweight, you are automatically at higher risk for some of today's most serious health problems. Centrally located (abdominal) fat, in particular, can lead to such conditions as heart disease, diabetes, high blood pressure, gout, gallstones, sleep apnea (snoring) and arthritis. It is thought that even if your fat is more uniformly distributed, it may affect your health by limiting your physical mobility, creating strain and pain in your joints, causing you to puff and pant with any physical exertion.

Aside from the physical side effects of being overweight, there are an equal number of emotional and psychological consequences, too. Your weight may inhibit you from meeting people, reduce your self esteem, make you feel unattractive, stop you from going swimming, make shopping for clothes a nightmare, stop you from playing with your children or prevent you from playing sports. Truth is, the extra weight you're carrying around might keep you from participating in a good many other activities that you might find enjoyable if you were thinner.

It is worthwhile taking control over aspects of your lifestyle that have an impact on your weight. You may not create a new body from your efforts, but you will feel better about the body you've got. Eating and exercising for your best performance is the aim of the game.

MEASURING THE FUEL WE NEED

Remember, calories are a measure of the fuel we need. Our bodies need a certain number of calories every day to work, just as a car needs so many gallons of gasoline to be driven a certain distance. Food and drink are our source of calories. If we eat and drink too much, we may store the extra calories as body fat. If we consume fewer calories than we need, our bodies will break down its stores of fat to make up for the shortfall.

WHAT WE REALLY NEED TO EAT
FOR HEALTH AND GROWTH

Food is part of our culture and way of life. Our food choices are determined by many factors ranging from religious beliefs to the deliciously sensual role that food plays in our lives. For babies, food has a comforting role to play, beyond meeting the immediate physical need. For adults, food reflects status—we prepare special meals for special occasions and for special guests to show respect or friendship.

It is no wonder that with so many factors influencing our food choices, we tend to overlook the very basic role food plays in the nourishment and growth of our bodies. In a busy lifestyle, it's easy to see food simply as a solution to overcoming hunger. In other circumstances, we focus on the social aspects of food and eat too much.

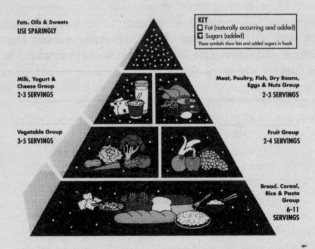

Source: United States Department of Agriculture and United States Department of Health and Human Services

In 1992, the United States Department of Agriculture (USDA) developed the Food Guide Pyramid, a food model that guides us on the types and amounts of foods we should be eating daily for health. For many reasons, our eating habits today fall very short of these recommendations.

Calorie-laden foods (sometimes called energy dense foods), such as alcohol, chocolate, potato chips and candy, provide few nutrients for a lot of calories. For this reason they are best limited to no more than one or two servings per day.

CUT THE FAT

So, our first message is to reduce the amount of fat you eat. This applies to all sorts of fat: saturated, polyunsaturated, monounsaturated. (Caution: A low fat diet is good for most of us, but it isn't appropriate for children who rely on fat for growth) But the flip side of this message is to eat more carbohydrate because doing so can help reduce your fat intake. The following chapters tell you how you can eat more carbohydrate and which foods you should choose to replace fatty foods. We also go one step further and tell you which carbohydrates are best for health—and why.

IT'S TIME TO TAKE CONTROL

It's never too late to make improvements in your health and lifestyle, so what better time to start than *right now*? You'll not only become fitter and healthier, but you'll also feel much better about the body you were born with.

Chapter 5

FACTORS THAT INFLUENCE BODY WEIGHT

WHAT'S INVOLVED

YOUR FAMILY TREE

HOW FAST YOUR MOTOR RUNS

*L*ike most health conditions, there are many different causes for being overweight, some of which include our genetic makeup, hormone levels, environmental factors, psychological issues and metabolic considerations.

For most of us, even without much conscious effort, our bodies maintain a relatively constant weight, often despite huge variations in how much we eat. For a proportion of people who are overweight, this apparent balancing of energy intake and output seems lost or inoperative. So, despite every fad diet, every exercise program, even operations and medications, body weight can steadily increase over the years, regardless of all apparent efforts to control it.

It has always been said that our weight is a result of how much we consume in relation to how much we burn up. So, if we take in too much (overeat) and don't burn up enough (don't exercise) we are likely to put on weight.

The question is: how much, of what, is too much?

The answer is not a simple one: Not all foods that we eat are equal and no two bodies are the same, given the wide variety of special factors we've outlined above.

WHAT'S INVOLVED

As we mentioned earlier, people are overweight for many different reasons. Some people believe they gain weight just from looking at food, while others say they have only to walk past a bakery to pack on a few extra pounds. Still other folks blame themselves because they eat too much. It is clear that a combination of social, genetic, dietary, metabolic, psychological (and emotional) factors combine to influence our weight. We've explained many of them below and in the next chapter.

- **Genetic predisposition.** Does excess weight run in your family?
- **Resting metabolic rate.** How much fuel does your body burn at rest?
- **Total food intake.** Do you eat too much food?
- **The balance of different nutrients.** Do you eat a healthy, balanced diet?
- **Energy expenditure associated with movement.** How much do you move in a normal day?
- **Thermic response to food.** How much fuel does your body waste as heat?

- **A body's preference to store excess calories as either fat or muscle.** Do you have more fat or muscle?
- **Energy expenditure associated with physical activity.** How much planned activity do you do?

YOUR FAMILY TREE

There are many overweight people who tell us resignedly that:

- "My mother/father is overweight, too."
- "I've always weighed too much."
- "It must be genetic."

Research shows us that these comments have much truth behind them. A child born to overweight parents is much more likely to be overweight than one whose parents were not overweight. It may sound like an excuse, but studies in twins provide evidence that our body weight and shape are at least partially determined by our genes.

Identical twins tend to be similar in body weight even if they are raised apart. Even twins adopted as infants show the body-fat profile of their true parents rather than that of their adoptive parents. These findings suggest that our genes are a stronger determinant of weight than our environment, which includes the food we eat.

How do genes play a role? It seems that information stored in our genes governs our tendency to store calories as either fat or as lean muscle tissue. Overfeeding a large group of identical twins confirmed that within each pair, weight gain was similar. The amount of weight gained between sets of identical twins varied greatly, however. From this, researchers concluded that our genes control the way our bodies respond to overeating. Some sets of twins gained a lot of weight, while others gained only a little, even though all were consuming an equivalent amount of excess calories.

All this isn't to say that if your parents were overweight, you should resign yourself to being overweight. But it may help you understand why you have to watch your weight while other people seemingly don't have to watch theirs.

So, if you were born with a tendency to be overweight, why does it matter what you eat? The answer is that foods (or more correctly, nutrients) are not equal in their effects on body weight. In particular, the way the body responds to dietary fat makes matters worse. If you're overweight, it is likely that the amount of fat you burn is small, relative to the amount of fat you store. Consequently, the more fat you eat, the more fat you store. Although this may sound logical, the "eat-more, store-more" mechanism does not exist for all nutrients.

Among all four major sources of calories in food, (protein, fat, carbohydrate and alcohol), fat is unique. When we increase our intake of protein, alcohol or carbohydrate, the body's response is to burn more of that particular energy source. Sensibly, the body matches the supply of fuel with the type of fuel burned. A fundamental difference between fat and carbohydrate is that fat tends to be stored, whereas carbohydrate has a tendency to be burned. If your carbohydrate intake is low, it may reduce the amount of calories you burn each day by 5 to 10 percent!

While you may not have been born owning the best set of genes for the current environment, you can still influence your weight by the lifestyle choices you make.

The message is simply this: If you believe that you are at risk of being overweight, you should think seriously about minimizing fat and eating more carbohydrate.

IT'S NOT JUST GENETICS

Despite a genetic predisposition, you can only gain weight if you take in more energy than you use. We know that obesity has many causes—for example, eating too much, exercising too little, genetics, aging, eating a high fat diet—all play a part. But what it all boils down to is that if we take in too much (overeat) and don't burn up enough (don't exercise) we are likely to put on weight.

HOW FAST YOUR MOTOR RUNS

Our genetic makeup also underlies our metabolism, which is basically how many calories we burn per minute. Bodies, like cars, differ in this regard. A V-8 consumes more fuel to run than a small four-cylinder car. A bigger body usually requires more calories than a smaller one.

Everyone has a resting metabolic rate, which is a measure of the amount of calories our bodies use when we are at rest. When a car is stationary, the engine idles—using just enough fuel to keep the motor running. When we are asleep, our engine keeps running, too (for example, our heart keeps beating) and we use a minimum number of calories. This is our basal metabolic rate.

When we start exercising, or even just moving around, the number of calories, or the amount of fuel we use, increases. However, the largest amount (around 70 percent) of the calories used in a 24-hour period, are those used to maintain our basic body functioning.

Since our resting metabolic rate is where most of the calories we eat are used, it is a significant determinant of our body weight. The lower your resting energy expenditure, the greater your risk of gaining weight, and vice versa.

Chapter 6

FOOD AND BODY BASICS

*I*t was widely (and wrongly) believed for many years that sugar and starchy foods such as potato, rice and pasta were the cause of obesity. Twenty years ago, every diet for weight loss advocated restriction of these carbohydrate-rich foods. One of the reasons for this carbohydrate restriction stemmed from the "instant results" of low carbohydrate diets. If your diet is very low in carbohydrate, you will lose weight. The problem is that what you primarily lose is fluid, and not fat. What's more, a low carbohydrate diet depletes the glycogen stores in the muscles thus making exercise difficult and tiring.

THE LOWDOWN ON SUGAR

Sugar has been blamed as a cause of excess weight primarily because it is often found in high fat foods, where it serves to make the fat more palatable and tempting. Chocolate, which contains almost one-third of its weight in the form of fat, would be fairly unpalatable without the sugar.

Current thinking is that there is little evidence to condemn sugar or starchy foods as the cause of excess weight. Overweight people show a preference for fat-containing foods rather than a preference for foods high in sugar. In a survey performed at the University of Michigan where obese men and women listed their favorite foods, men listed mainly meats (protein-fat sources) and women listed mainly cakes, cookies, doughnuts (combinations of carbohydrate and fat sources). Other studies have found that obese people habitually consume a higher fat diet than people who have a healthy weight. So, it appears that a higher intake of fatty food is strongly related to the development of obesity—not carbohydrate-rich foods.

COUNTING THE CALORIES
IN OUR NUTRIENTS

All foods contain calories. Often the caloric content of a food is considered a measure of how fattening it is. Of all the nutrients in food that we consume, carbohydrate yields the fewest calories per gram.

carbohydrate	4 calories per gram
protein	4 calories per gram

alcohol	7 calories per gram
fat	9 calories per gram

Whether you are going to gain weight from eating a particular food really depends on how much that food adds to your total calorie intake in relation to how much you burn up.

To lose weight you need to eat fewer calories and burn more calories. If your total calorie balance does not change—there will be no change in your weight. People who consume a high fat diet tend to eat a high calorie diet, because fatty foods yield more calories for the same weight of food than carbohydrate foods. (This is why substituting low fat foods for high fat foods and a focus on reducing your total fat intake has the most potential to reduce your calorie intake.)

DID YOU KNOW?

Our bodies love to store fat, since that extra "insulation" will help protect us in case of famine. So, even in the midst of plenty we're building up our fat reserves!

WHICH FOODS ARE MOST FATTENING?

Let's compare two everyday foods that are almost "pure" in a nutritional sense.

3 teaspoons of sugar	versus	1 teaspoon of butter
(almost pure carbohydrate)		(almost pure fat)

They contain virtually the same number of calories.

46 calories   versus   45 calories

This means that you can eat three times the volume of sugar as you could butter for the same number of calories! Look at these other examples:

- A small grilled T-bone steak (about the size of a slice of bread) has the same calories as 3 medium potatoes.
- 3 slices of bread, thickly buttered, are equivalent to 6 slices of bread with no butter.
- 4 Oreos have more calories than a carton of 2% chocolate milk.
- Eating 1 piece of breaded, fried chicken at lunch is the caloric equivalent of 6 slices of bread (without butter).
- For every 1 cup of fried rice you eat you could eat 2 cups of boiled rice
- And if you're feeling extra hungry next time you stop for a coffee, consider that 1 glazed doughnut has the calories of 3 slices of lightly buttered cinnamon-raisin toast!

In every case the highest fat foods have the highest calorie counts. Because carbohydrate has about half the calories of fat, it is safer to eat more carbohydrate-rich food. What's more, your body is more likely to store fat and burn carbohydrate so the calories contribute more to your "spread" when they come from fat.

■ ■ ■

ARE YOU REALLY CHOOSING LOW FAT?

There's a trick to food labels that it is worth being aware of when shopping for low fat foods. These food labeling specifications guidelines were enacted by the United States Department of Agriculture (USDA) in 1994:

Free: Contains a tiny or insignificant amount of fat, cholesterol, sodium, sugar or calories; less than 0.5 grams (g) of fat per serving.

Low fat: Contains no more than 3 g of fat per serving.

Reduced/Less/Fewer: These diet products must contain 25% less of a nutrient to calories than the regular product.

Light/Lite: These diet products contain ⅓ fewer calories than, or ½ the fat of, the original product.

Lean: Meats with "lean" on the label contain less than 10 g of fat, 4 g of saturated fat, and 95 milligrams (mg) of cholesterol per serving.

Extra lean: These meats have less than 5 g of fat, 2 g of saturated fat and 95 mg of cholesterol per serving.

■

A GNAWING, EMPTY FEELING
ISN'T NECESSARY WHEN YOU ARE
LOSING WEIGHT BECAUSE LOW
G.I. FOODS ARE FILLING AND
PREVENT HUNGER PANGS FOR LONGER.

■

FOUR FOOD TIPS TO HELP YOU LOSE WEIGHT

1. Eat regular meals—include between-meal snacks if you're hungry.
2. Try to include a low G.I. food at every meal.
3. Ensure that your meals contain mainly carbohydrate and only a little fat.
4. Eat low carbohydrate foods such as carrots, broccoli and salads freely, but don't eat them instead of the high carbohydrate foods.

■

CARBOHYDRATES ARE NATURAL APPETITE
SUPPRESSANTS. AND OF ALL CARBOHYDRATE
FOODS, THOSE WITH A LOW GLYCEMIC INDEX
ARE AMONG THE MOST FILLING AND
PREVENT HUNGER PANGS FOR LONGER.

■

Chapter 7

EXERCISE: WE CAN'T LIVE WITHOUT IT

THE BENEFITS OF EXERCISE

HOW TO GET MOVING

8 WAYS TO MAKE EXERCISE WORK FOR YOU

A multitude of changes in living habits now mean that in both work and recreation we are more sedentary. Our physical activity levels are now so low that we have an imbalance in our energy equation so that we don't burn up enough calories to account for the amount we eat.

■

TO LOSE WEIGHT YOU NEED TO EAT FEWER CALORIES AND BURN MORE CALORIES——AND THAT MEANS GETTING REGULAR EXERCISE AND LEADING A MORE ACTIVE LIFESTYLE.

■

THE BENEFITS OF EXERCISE

Most people could tell you at least one health benefit of exercise (reduces blood pressure, lowers the risk of heart disease, improves circulation, increases stamina, flexibility and strength), but the most motivating aspect of exercise is feeling so good about yourself for doing it.

Exercise speeds up our metabolic rate. By increasing our caloric expenditure, exercise helps to balance our sometimes excessive caloric intake from food.

More movement makes our muscles better at using fat as a source of fuel. By improving the way insulin works, exercise increases the amount of fat we burn.

A low G.I. diet has the same effect. Low G.I. foods reduce the amount of insulin we need, which makes fat easier to burn and harder to store. Since it's body fat that you want to get rid of when you lose weight, exercise in combination with a low G.I. diet makes a lot of sense!

HOW TO GET MOVING

Getting more exercise doesn't necessarily mean daily aerobics classes and jogging around the block (although this is great if you want to do it). What it *does* mean is moving more in everyday living. It's the day-to-day things we do—shopping, ironing, chasing kids, walking from the train station—where we spend the bulk of our energy. Since so much of our lifestyle is designed now to reduce our physical exertion, it's become very important to catch bursts of physical activity wherever we can, to increase our energy output. It may mean using the stairs instead of the elevator, taking a 10-minute walk at lunch time, trotting on a treadmill while you watch the news or talk on the telephone, walking to the grocery store to get the Sunday paper, hiding the remote control, parking a half mile from work or taking the dog for a walk each night. Whatever it means, do it. Even housework burns calories!

HOW EXERCISE KEEPS YOU MOVING

The effect of exercise doesn't stop when you do. People who exercise have higher metabolic rates, so their bodies continue to burn more calories every minute, even when they're asleep!

Besides increasing the incidental activity you will also benefit from some planned aerobic activity, which causes you to breathe more heavily and makes your heart beat faster. Walking, cycling, swimming and stair climbing are just a few examples. You'll need to accumulate a total of at least 30 minutes of this type of activity five to six days a week.

Remember that reduction in body weight takes time. Even after you've made changes in your exercise habits, your weight may not be any different on the scales. This is particularly true in women, whose bodies tend to adapt to increased caloric expenditure.

Whatever it takes for you to burn more calories, do it. Try to regard movement as an opportunity to improve your physical well being—not as an inconvenience.

8 WAYS TO MAKE EXERCISE WORK FOR YOU

Your exercise routine will bring you lots of benefits if you can:

1. see how it benefits you
2. enjoy what you do
3. feel that you can do it fairly well
4. fit it in with your daily life
5. keep it inexpensive
6. make it accessible
7. stay safe while doing it
8. make it socially acceptable to your peers

■

EXERCISE MAKES OUR
MUSCLES BETTER AT USING
FAT AS A SOURCE OF FUEL.

■

Chapter 8

DO YOU GET ALL THE NUTRIENTS YOU NEED?

BREADS/CEREALS/GRAINS

VEGETABLES

FRUIT

DAIRY FOODS

MEAT AND ALTERNATIVES

To meet your average daily nutrient requirements you need to eat a certain amount of different types of foods. If you are trying to reduce your caloric intake there is still a minimum amount of certain foods that you should be eating each day. These are:

BREADS/CEREALS/AND GRAIN FOODS —6 SERVINGS OR MORE

1 serving means:
- 1 bowl breakfast cereal (1 ounce)
- ½ cup cooked pasta or rice

- ½ cup cooked grain such as barley or wheat
- 1 slice bread
- ½ roll or muffin

VEGETABLES—3 SERVINGS

1 serving means:
- 1 medium potato (about 5 ounces)
- ½ cup cooked vegetables such as broccoli or carrot (2 ounces)
- 1 cup raw leafy vegetables, such as lettuce

FRUIT—2–4 SERVINGS

1 serving means:
- 1 medium orange (7 ounces)
- 1 medium apple (5 ounces)
- ½ cup strawberries (4 ounces)

DAIRY FOODS—2 SERVINGS

1 serving means:
- 8 ounces low fat milk
- 1½ ounces low fat cheese
- 8 ounces low fat yogurt

MEAT AND ALTERNATIVES—2 SERVINGS

1 serving means:
- 3 ounces cooked lean beef, veal, lamb or pork
- 3 ounces lean chicken (cooked, excluding bone)

- 3 ounces fish (cooked, excluding bone)
- 2 eggs
- ½ cup cooked beans

If you prefer larger servings of meat, go ahead, just make sure it's lean. Protein is a very satiating nutrient.

Chapter 9

HOW WELL ARE YOU EATING NOW?

DO YOU EAT ENOUGH CARBOHYDRATE?

IS YOUR DIET TOO HIGH IN FAT?

HOW DID YOU RATE?

---

*Y*ou can check the nutritional quality of your diet yourself; all you need is a record of your usual food intake. It is ideal if you can keep a food diary of everything you eat and drink for three to five days and use this for your assessment. Remember, you have to eat as freely as you normally do and write down everything—otherwise you're only cheating yourself!

Once you have your total food intake record complete, use the serving size guidelines in the charts below to check whether you have a balanced intake. The checklists on the following pages can be used to assess your carbohydrate and fat intake.

LOW G.I. EATING

Low G.I. eating means making a move back to the high carbohydrate foods that are staples in many parts of the world, especially whole grains (barley, oats, dried peas and beans) in combination with breads, pasta, vegetables, fruits and certain types of rice.

DO YOU EAT ENOUGH CARBOHYDRATE?

Looking at your diet record and using the serving size guide below estimate the number of servings of carbohydrate foods you had each day. For example, if you had a banana, 2 slices of bread and a medium potato, this counts as 4 servings of carbohydrate.

CARBOHYDRATE FOOD	ONE SERVING IS	HOW MANY DID YOU EAT?
Fruit	a handful or 1 medium piece	
Juice	about ¾ cup (6 ozs.)	
Dried fruit	¼ cup	
Bread	1 slice	
English muffin, bread, roll, bagel	½ roll, muffin or small bagel	
Crackers, crispbread	2 large pieces or 3-4 plain crackers	
Rice cakes	2 rice cakes	
Muffin, cookies	½ muffin or 2 cookies	
Health bar/sports bar	approximately ½ average bar	
Breakfast cereal	1 bowl (1 oz.)	
Oatmeal	about ½ cup cooked cereal	
Rice	½ cup cooked rice	

CARBOHYDRATE FOOD	ONE SERVING IS	HOW MANY DID YOU EAT?
Pasta, noodles	½ cup cooked noodles	
Pancakes	1 pancake, 4 inch	
Bulgur, couscous	about ⅓ cup, cooked	
Potato, sweet potato	1 small potato, about 3 ozs.	
Sweet corn	1 small ear or ½ cup kernels	
Lentils	½ cup, cooked	
Baked beans, other beans	about ½ cup, cooked	
Total		

Average the number of servings over all the days to come up with a daily average.

HOW DID YOU RATE?

- **Less than 4 servings a day:** Poor.
- **Between 4 and 8 servings a day:** Fair, but you need to eat a lot more.
- **Between 9 and 12 servings a day:** Good, could need more if you are hungry.
- **Between 13 and 16 servings a day:** Great—this should meet the needs of most people.

IS YOUR DIET TOO HIGH IN FAT?

Use this fat counter to tally up how much fat your diet contains. Do a tally for each day and then take an average. Using this fat counter you will need to compare the serving size listed with your serving size and multiply the grams of fat up or down to match your serving size. For example, if you estimate you might consume 2 cups of regular milk in a day, this supplies you with 16 grams of fat.

FOOD	FAT CONTENT (GRAMS)	HOW MUCH DID YOU EAT?
Dairy Foods		
Milk, (8 ozs.) 1 cup		
whole	8	
2%	5	
nonfat	0	
Yogurt, (8 ozs.)		
whole milk	7	
nonfat	0	
Ice cream, 2 scoops, (1 cup)		
regular	15	
low fat	3	
fat free	0	
Cheese		
American, block cheese, 1 oz. slice	9	
reduced fat American cheese, 1 oz. slice	7	
low fat slices (per slice)	3	
cottage, small curd, 2 tablespoons	3	
ricotta, whole milk, 2 tablespoons	2	
Cream, 1 tablespoon		
heavy	6	
light	5	
Sour cream, 1 tablespoon		
regular	3	
light	1	
Fats and Oils		
Butter, 1 teaspoon	4	
Oil, any type, 1 tablespoon, (½ oz.)	14	
Cooking spray, per spray	0	
Mayonnaise, 1 tablespoon	11	
Salad dressing, 1 tablespoon	6	

FOOD	FAT CONTENT (GRAMS)	HOW MUCH DID YOU EAT?
Meat		
Beef		
steak, flank, lean only, 3½ ozs.	10	
ground beef, extra-lean, 1 cup, 3½ ozs., cooked, drained	16	
sausage, frankfurter, grilled, 2 ozs.	16	
top sirloin, lean only, 3½ ozs.	8	
Lamb		
rib chop, grilled, lean only, 3½ ozs.	10	
leg, roasted, lean only, 3½ ozs.	7	
loin chop, grilled, lean only, 3 ½ ozs.	8	
Pork		
bacon, 3 strips, panfried	9	
ham, 1 slice, leg, lean, 3½ ozs.	5	
steak, lean only, 3½ ozs.	4	
leg, roasted, lean only, 3½ ozs.	9	
loin chop, lean only, 3½ ozs.	4	
Chicken		
breast, skinless, 3 ozs.	4	
drumstick, skinless, 2 ozs.	3	
thigh, skinless, 2 ozs.	6	
½ barbecue chicken (including skin)	30	
Fish		
grilled fish, 1 average fillet, 4 ozs.	1	
salmon, 3 ozs.	3	
fish sticks, frozen, 4 baked	14	
fish fillets, 2, batter-dipped, frozen, oven-baked, 6 ozs.		
regular	26	
light	10	
Snack Foods		
Chocolate bar, Hershey, 1½ ozs.	13	
Potato chips, 1 oz. bag	10	

FOOD	FAT CONTENT (GRAMS)	HOW MUCH DID YOU EAT?
Corn chips, 1 oz. bag	10	
Peanuts, ½ cup, (2½ ozs.)	35	
French fries, 25 pieces	20	
Pizza, cheese, 2 slices, medium pizza	22	
Pie, apple, snack size	15	
Popcorn, fat and salt added, 3 cups	9	
Total		

HOW DID YOU RATE?

- **Less than 40 grams:** Excellent. Thirty to 40 grams of fat per day is recommended for those people trying to lose weight.
- **41 to 60 grams:** Good. A fat intake in this range is recommended for most adult men and women.
- **61 to 80 grams:** Acceptable if you are very active (doing hard physical work or athletic training). It is probably too much if you are trying to lose weight.
- **More than 80 grams:** You're probably eating too much fat, unless you're Superman or Superwoman!

Chapter 10

A LOW G.I. DIET MADE EASY

7 QUICK LOW FAT, LOW G.I. BREAKFAST IDEAS

9 LOW G.I. LUNCHES ON THE GO

7 LOW G.I. DINNER IDEAS

7 QUICK AND EASY LOW G.I. DESSERTS

Once you know how to eat the low G.I. way and which foods to reach for when you're hungry, it's easy to prepare low fat, low G.I. meals any time of the day. Here are a few ideas to get you started.

BREAKFAST

- Start with a bowl of low G.I. cereal served with skim or 1% milk or yogurt.
- Try a bowl of All-Bran or rolled oats (raw or cooked).
- If you prefer muesli or granola, keep to a small

bowl of a low fat version—check that it doesn't contain added fat.

- Add a slice of toast made from 100% stoneground whole wheat bread or whole grain pumpernickel (or 2 slices for a bigger person) with a tablespoon of jam, sliced banana, honey, marmalade or light cream cheese with sliced apple. Keep butter to a minimum, or use none at all.
- If you like a hot breakfast, try a boiled or poached egg with your toast.

7 quick low fat, low G.I. breakfast ideas

1. Spread raisin toast with light cream cheese and top with sliced apple.
2. Toast stoneground whole wheat bread and top with sliced banana.
3. Make old-fashioned oats with 1% milk; sprinkle with raisins and brown sugar.
4. Whip up a fruit smoothie with 1% milk, yogurt, banana and honey.
5. Top one 8 ounce container of light yogurt with sliced peaches and raspberries.
6. Try a bowl of All-Bran, with 1% milk and unsweetened canned pear slices.
7. Enjoy a sourdough English muffin with natural peanut butter and spreadable fruit.

LUNCH

- Try a sandwich or roll, with only a dab of butter. Choose 100% stoneground whole wheat, whole grain pumpernickel or any other bread made with lots of whole grains. Add plenty of sliced vegetables.

- For the filling, choose from a thin slice of ham, pastrami, lean roast beef or chicken or turkey breast, or a slice of low fat cheese, salmon or tuna (in water) or an egg. An extra container of salad or vegetable soup will help to fill you up.
- Finish your lunch with a piece of fruit, fruit salad with a low fat yogurt or a low fat chocolate or plain milk.

9 low G.I. lunches on the go

1. Take some pita bread, spread it with hummus and fill with tabouli.
2. Enjoy some chunky vegetable soup, thick with barley, beans and noodles.
3. Cook a little pasta and mix with pesto, sundried tomatoes or chopped fresh herbs and olive oil.
4. Put your favorite sandwich filling on dark rye bread (you can grill the sandwich if you like).
5. In a blender, whip up a banana smoothie and couple it with a high-fiber apple muffin.
6. Mix fresh fruit with nonfat yogurt.
7. Microwave a potato. Split it open and top with baked beans and a sprinkle of grated cheese. (Don't forget to eat the skin!)
8. Steam or microwave an ear of fresh corn and enjoy as is. Finish with some fruit and yogurt.
9. Couple a green salad with some bean salad, add whole grain bread and enjoy.

DINNER

- The basis of dinner should be carbohydrate foods. Take your pick from rice, pasta, potato, sweet potato, couscous, bread, legumes or a mixture.

- Then, add as many vegetables as you can, using a small amount of meat, chicken or fish as a flavoring, rather than the main ingredient.
- Use lean meat, such as London broil, veal, center cut pork chop, trimmed lamb, chicken breast, fish fillets or turkey. Red meat is a valuable source of iron—just choose lean types. A piece of meat, chicken or fish that fits in the palm of your hand is your proper protein portion for dinner.
- If you prefer not to eat meat, a cup of cooked dried peas, beans, lentils or chickpeas can provide protein and iron without any fat. At the same time they supply low G.I. carbohydrate and fiber.
- Vegetarian products such as veggie burgers, tempeh and tofu are based on high protein legumes (such as soybeans and peanuts) and are good meat alternatives.
- Boost your fruit intake and get into the habit of finishing your meal with fruit—fresh, stewed or baked. Or try a fruit ice, such as Dole Fruit Juice Bars.

7 low G.I. dinner ideas

1. Team a lean mix of Bolognese sauce (extra lean ground beef with onions, garlic, tomatoes, celery and carrots) with spaghetti and a green salad.
2. Stir-fry chicken, meat or fish with mixed green vegetables. Serve with Basmati rice or Chinese noodles.
3. Serve vegetable lasagna with salad.
4. Grill a steak and serve with a trio of low G.I. vegetables—new potato, sweet corn and peas.
5. Cook spinach and ricotta tortellini with garden

vegetables and a tomato and mushroom sauce.
6. Wrap a fish fillet dressed with lemon, parsley and garlic in foil. Bake and serve with mixed vegetables or salad.
7. Buy a barbecued chicken, steam sweet ears of corn and toss a salad together.

7 quick and easy low G.I. desserts

1. Top low fat ice cream with strawberries.
2. Stuff a whole apple with dried fruit and bake it.
3. Mix a fruit salad with low fat yogurt.
4. Fruit crisp: Top cooked fruit with a crumbled mixture of toasted muesli, wheat flakes, a little melted butter and honey.
5. Banana pudding: Slice a firm banana into some low fat pudding.
6. Fruited cream: Top canned fruit, such as peaches or pears with low fat ice cream, low fat pudding or sugar free Jell-O.
7. Fruit strudel: Wrap chopped apple, raisins, currants and spice in a sheet of filo pastry (brushed with milk, not fat) and bake as a strudel.

G.I. RANGES

Low G.I. Foods	below 55
Intermediate G.I. Foods	between 55 and 70
High G.I. Foods	more than 70

Chapter 11

SECRETS TO LOW G.I. SNACKING

5 SNACKING TIPS

17 SUSTAINING SNACKS

*I*t's normal to get hungry and want to snack between your usual "three squares." Luckily, when you eat the low G.I. way there's no prohibition on between-meal nibbles. It's a great way to eat the foods you love without gaining weight!

Just remember that when you choose a between-meal bite, pick a low fat snack with a low glycemic index. For example, an apple with a glycemic index of 38 is better than a slice of white bread with a glycemic index of around 70, and will result in a smaller blood sugar jump.

New evidence suggests that the people who graze, eating small amounts of food throughout the day at frequent intervals, may actually be doing themselves a favor. Spreading the food out over longer periods of time will flatten out the peaks and valleys of blood glucose levels. So, snacking may be a good idea—as long as you don't overeat and gain weight.

Some snack foods with low G.I. values (such as peanuts, at 14) have a very high fat content and are not recommended for people trying to lose weight. As an occasional snack they are fine, especially because their fat is the healthier monounsaturated type. Just don't indulge in them every day. Remember, with peanuts, it's often hard to stop at just a handful!

5 SNACKING TIPS

- It is important to include a couple of servings of dairy foods each day for your calcium needs. If you haven't used yogurt or cheese in any meals, you may choose to make a low fat milkshake. One or 2 scoops of low fat ice cream or pudding can also boost your daily calcium intake.
- If you like whole grain breads, an extra slice makes a very good choice for a snack. Other snacks can include toasted sourdough English muffin halves, a waffle or a slice of raisin bread with a little butter.
- Fruit is always a low calorie option for snacks. You should try to consume at least 3 servings a day. It may be helpful to prepare fruit in advance to make it accessible and easy to eat.
- Ryvita whole grain crispbreads are a low calorie snack if you want something dry and crunchy. Popcorn (prepared at home using a minimum of fat) is another good alternative.

- Keep vegetables (such as celery and carrot sticks, baby tomatoes, florets of blanched cauliflower or broccoli) ready prepared.

SNACKING SUCCESS!

A recent study that compared people eating a diet of three meals a day with those who had three meals and three snacks showed that snacking stimulated the body to use up more energy for metabolism compared with concentrating the same amount of food into three meals. It's as if the more fuel you give your body the more it will burn. Frequent small meals stimulate the metabolic rate.

---

17 SUSTAINING SNACKS

- An apple
- An apple and oat bran muffin
- Dried apricots
- A mini can of baked beans
- A small bowl of cherries
- Ice cream (low fat) in a cone
- Milk, milkshake or smoothie (low fat, of course)
- Oatmeal cookies, 2 to 3
- An orange
- Six ounces of orange juice, freshly squeezed
- Pita bread spread with apple butter
- A big bowl of low fat popcorn
- One or 2 slices of raisin toast
- Whole grain bread sandwich with your favorite filling
- A bowl of Raisin Bran™ with skim milk
- A small box of raisins
- Six to 8 ounces of light yogurt

Chapter 12

THE LOW G.I. PANTRY

BREADS

BREAKFAST CEREALS

RICE AND GRAINS

LEGUMES

VEGETABLES

FRUITS

DAIRY FOODS

USEFUL FLAVORINGS, SAUCES
AND DRESSINGS

To make low G.I. choices easier, you need to keep the right foods in your cupboard and refrigerator. Here's a starter list for you to follow.

BREADS

If you're the only one in the house who will eat the "birdseed bread," keep a loaf in the freezer and pull out slices as you need them.

- 100% stoneground whole wheat
- Arnold's rye
- Banana bread

- Chapati (baisen)
- Natural Ovens 100% Whole Grain
- Natural Ovens Happiness
- Natural Ovens Hunger Filler
- Natural Ovens Natural Wheat
- Sourdough
- Sourdough rye
- Whole grain pumpernickel
- Whole wheat pita

Natural Ovens breads are available in the United States through mail order. See "For More Information" on page 112 for ordering information.

BREAKFAST CEREALS

- Kellogg's All-Bran with Extra Fiber™
- Kellogg's Bran Buds with Psyllium™
- Muesli (low fat varieties, read the labels)
- Rolled or old-fashioned oats
- Oat bran
- Rice bran
- Oatmeal

RICE AND GRAINS

- Pearled barley
- Basmati rice, brown or long grain rice
- Uncle Ben's Converted™ Rice
- Pasta of various shapes and flavors

LEGUMES

- Cooked lentils (red or brown), chickpeas, split peas
- Dried lentils, chickpeas, cannellini beans
- A variety of canned legumes (kidney beans, mixed beans, baked beans, lentils, chickpeas, black beans, pinto beans, butter beans, broad beans, chana dal)

VEGETABLES

- Peas
- Sweet corn
- Sweet potato
- Canned new potatoes
- Carrots

Other canned vegetables such as tomatoes, asparagus, peas and mushrooms are handy to boost the vegetable content of a meal. Other convenient products are:

- Tomato paste
- Tomato puree
- Bottled tomato pasta sauces
- Frozen vegetables

FRUITS

- Cherries
- Grapefruit
- Pears
- Apples

- Plums
- Peaches
- Oranges
- Grapes
- Kiwi
- Dried fruits, such as dried apricots, fruit medley, raisins, prunes etc.
- Canned peaches, pears, apple as a useful stand-by
- Frozen berries and melon balls

DAIRY FOODS

- Yogurt—low fat, fruited and plain
- 1% or skim milk
- Shelf-stable skim milk or skim milk powder—easy to use in cooking
- Canned evaporated skim milk
- Cook 'n' Serve Sugar Free Pudding and Pie Filling
- Low fat ice cream
- Frozen low fat yogurt, sorbet, gelato
- Eggs

Cheese
- Low fat processed slices
- Reduced fat Swiss (such as Jarlsberg Light)
- Grated parmesan
- 1% or 2% cottage or part skim ricotta cheese

USEFUL FLAVORINGS, SAUCES AND DRESSINGS

- Spices—curry powder, cumin, turmeric, mustard etc.

- Herbs—oregano, basil, thyme etc.
- Bottled minced ginger, chili and garlic
- Sauces (such as soy, chili, oyster, hoi sin, teriyaki, Worcestershire)
- Bouillon
- Low oil salad dressings

■

IN OUR EXPERIENCE, LOOKING AT THE DIETS OF PEOPLE
WHO WANT TO LOSE WEIGHT, THE CHANGE REQUIRED
IS OFTEN TO EAT MORE.

■

Chapter 13

7 DAYS OF LOW G.I. MEALS

*H*ere's a whole week of healthy, low calorie menus with all the benefits of low G.I. foods. Each menu is designed to be:

- **low in fat.** Eating less fat is an easy way to reduce your energy intake. To lose weight we recommend aiming for a daily fat intake of 30 to 50 g. We've used skim or 1% milk and minimal added fat throughout the menus.
- **high in carbohydrate with a low glycemic index.** Carbohydrates, especially those with a low glycemic index, are the most satisfying for your appetite. It's also the best fuel for your body so we've made sure that at least half the calories each day come from carbohydrate. This means

eating around 200 g a day as a minimum.
- **low in calories.** You'll lose weight if you reduce your calorie intake, but it's important not to go too low. We've aimed for a daily average of 1200 to 1400 calories.
- **nutritionally balanced.** Including a large variety of foods, but in the right proportions, makes you more likely to meet your nutrient needs.

These menus are not a prescription! Use them for ideas and as a guide to the amounts and types of foods for a low calorie diet.

10 TIPS TO CONTROL YOUR FOOD INTAKE

- Use hunger as the cue for eating—not the time of day.
- Eat a low G.I. carbohydrate food when you are hungry— these foods are the most satiating.
- Slow down when you eat to give your stomach a chance to give the signal to your brain that it is full.
- When you are thinking about eating, ask yourself how hungry you really are. Delay eating for 30 minutes—true hunger will return.
- Don't buy the foods that you don't want to eat.
- Indulge in the occasional treat. Lollipops or hard candies are more filling than chocolates.
- Give yourself time to make changes in your habits. It takes about 6 weeks for your tastebuds to readjust.
- Once you have served your meal or snack, put the remaining food away, so it is out of sight.
- Keep busy during the day.
- Don't restrain your food intake excessively—use the eating checklists in Chapter 9 (pages 42–50) to make sure you eat enough.

MONDAY

G.I.:	49
TOTAL ENERGY:	1474 cal.
FAT:	34 g
CARBOHYDRATE:	232 g
FIBER:	32 g

Breakfast:
Oatmeal and fruit

Cook or microwave a bowl of oatmeal using ½ cup old-fashioned oats. Top with 8 ounces milk, 1 tablespoon sugar and serve with a 4 ounce glass of orange juice.

Alternative:
Soften the oats for a little while in cold 1% milk and eat them as muesli, topped with a sliced banana.

Morning snack:
Eight dried apricot halves and a cup of lemon tea or coffee

Lunch:
Ham and salad sandwich

Make a ham sandwich with 2 slices of 100% stoneground whole wheat bread, 2 ounces boiled ham, lettuce, tomato, mustard, grated carrot and sprouts. Finish with a small juicy apple.

Afternoon snack:
Two oatmeal cookies and a cup of coffee

Dinner:
Vegetarian lasagna and salad

See *The Glucose Revolution* for our low fat, low G.I. recipe for Vegetarian Lasagna (p. 190). Serve with a side salad of your choice. For dessert, try a fresh fruit salad and a ½ cup scoop of low fat ice cream.

Evening snack:
Fun size Snickers (or other) chocolate bar

MARGARINE: FRIEND OR FOE?

You'll notice that in some of these meals, we suggest using light margarine. As you may know, many margarines are sources of trans fats, which can raise cholesterol levels and have been implicated in increased risk of heart attacks and possibly even breast cancer. Luckily, not all margarine is created equal! Some products now on store shelves clearly boast that they are trans-fat free (look for those). Here are some other guidelines Johanna Burani, M.S., R.D., C.D.E., suggests you follow to avoid these unhealthy fats:

- Buy margarine by the tub, not the stick
- Look for "light," "low fat," "nonfat" or "fat free" on the label
- Make sure the first ingredient says "liquid," such as "liquid corn oil" or "liquid safflower oil"

TUESDAY

G.I.:	47
TOTAL ENERGY::	1543 cal.
FAT:	47 g
CARBOHYDRATE:	202 g
FIBER:	31 g

Breakfast:
Peanut butter toast
Top a slice of 100% stoneground whole wheat toast with 1 tablespoon natural peanut butter. Finish off with a pear or other fresh fruit.

Morning snack:
A small bunch of grapes

Lunch:
Soup and bread
Team a 1 cup bowl of split pea and ham soup with 3 stoneground wheat thins. Complete the meal with an orange.

Afternoon snack:
Enjoy an iced coffee, made with 8 ounces 1% milk

Dinner:
Spaghetti Bolognese
See our book *The Glucose Revolution* for a low fat, low G.I. Bolognese sauce recipe (p. 189) and serve ⅓ cup sauce over 1 cup cooked spaghetti. Accompany with a side salad.

Evening snack:
A small handful of peanuts (1 ounce). If you think you might have trouble sticking to this amount, make sure you buy peanuts in the shell—at least that will slow you down!

WEDNESDAY

G.I.:	53
TOTAL ENERGY:	1267 cal.
FAT:	19 g
CARBOHYDRATE:	202 g
FIBER:	32g

Breakfast:
Cereal and fruit
Two-thirds of a cup of All Bran with extra fiber,
topped with 6 ounces 1% milk. Add 4 unsweetened canned peaches to the cereal or accompany
with a 4 ounce glass of fruit juice.

Morning snack:
Handful of pretzels (about 10)

Lunch:
Pasta and sauce
Top a cup of boiled pasta with about ⅓ cup of bottled tomato and mushroom sauce. Add a tossed
green salad, drizzled with fat free dressing.

Afternoon snack:
Small scoop (½ cup) nonfat ice cream in a cup or
cone

Dinner:
Tuna casserole with rice
Make a quick tuna casserole using a 3 ounce can
of tuna, onion, celery and peas combined in a
cheese sauce. Serve with 1 cup Basmati or long
grain rice, seasoned with fresh parsley.

Evening snack:
A cup of fresh fruit salad

THURSDAY

G.I.:	48
TOTAL ENERGY:	1394 cal.
FAT:	38 g
CARBOHYDRATE:	90 g
FIBER:	23 g

Breakfast:
Muesli and yogurt
Pour 2 ounces nonfat milk over ½ cup natural muesli. Top with 4 ounces light fruited yogurt and 4 ounces fresh or unsweetened canned peaches.

Morning snack:
Two oatmeal cookies and a cup of tea or coffee

Lunch:
Toasted sandwich
Make a grilled cheese and tomato sandwich on toasted 100% stoneground whole wheat bread. Finish with a crunchy apple.

Afternoon snack:
Toast a slice of raisin bread and spread lightly with ½ tablespoon light margarine. Drink a cup of light, no-sugar-added hot chocolate with it.

Dinner:
Pork and vegetables
Grill or broil a 3 ounce center loin pork cutlet, basting with a favorite marinade if desired. Serve with 3 steamed new potatoes, a small ear of corn on the cob, ½ cup broccoli and ½ cup green beans.

Dessert:
Have ½ cup of canned peaches and 1 scoop of low fat ice cream and finish the meal with a cup of fla-vored decaf coffee.

FRIDAY

G.I.:	44
TOTAL ENERGY:	1385 cal.
FAT:	29 g
CARBOHYDRATE:	203 g
FIBER:	27 g

Breakfast:
Tea and toast
One half grapefruit with a teaspoon of sugar, followed by 2 slices of pumpernickel bread toast spread with 1 tablespoon light cream cheese and 1 ounce salmon. Finish with a cup of tea.

Morning snack:
A cup of sugar free hot chocolate

Lunch:
Stuffed potato and beans
Microwave a large (9 ounce) baking potato in its skin until tender. Cut off the top and fill with ⅓ cup baked beans and 1 tablespoon of grated cheese.

Afternoon snack:
An 8 ounce container of light yogurt

Alternative:
Fruit smoothie: Blend together a peach (or other seasonal fruit) with 4 ounces of light yogurt.

Dinner:
Beef stroganoff with mushrooms and wine
Small serving of casserole (containing approximately 3 ounces cubed tenderloin). Serve with 1 cup of boiled fettucine, ½ cup of green beans and baby carrots.

Evening snack:
Small bag (1 ounce) of potato chips

SATURDAY

G.I.:	45
TOTAL ENERGY:	1511 cal.
FAT:	31 g
CARBOHYDRATE:	216 g
FIBER:	23 g

Breakfast:
Egg and bagel
A hard or soft boiled egg and half a bagel topped
with 1 tablespoon light margarine. Finish with an
8 ounce cup of nonfat, no sugar added hot chocolate.

Morning snack:
Low fat honey 'n' oats granola bar

Lunch:
Vegetable grain toss
Mix 1 cup of a cooked commercial whole grain
mix (such as Lipton Rice and Sauce with Cajun
Style Beans, Casbah Wheat Pilaf or Near East
Barley Pilaf) with 1 cup of fresh or frozen cooked
vegetables. Toss.

Afternoon snack:
A small low fat ice cream cone

Dinner:
Lemon flounder with vegetables
Broil or poach 2 5-ounce flounder fillets in lemon
juice and white wine. Season with herbs and spices
as desired. Serve with a cup of boiled Basmati or
Uncle Ben's Converted Rice, ½ cup of steamed
broccoli and ½ cup of carrots.

Evening snack:
A large pear

SUNDAY

G.I.:	52
TOTAL ENERGY:	1294 cal.
FAT:	34 g
CARBOHYDRATE:	180 g
FIBER:	24 g

Breakfast:
Sunday smoothie
Blend ¾ cup of 1% milk, ¼ cup plain nonfat yogurt,
½ teaspoon honey, a small banana and a dash of nut-
meg in a blender, for a delicious, nourishing drink.

Morning snack:
A thin slice of banana bread with tea or coffee

Lunch:
Pita pizza
Toast 2 ounce whole wheat pita. With the bottom
side up, cover with tomato sauce, basil, oregano
and 2 ounces part skim shredded mozzarella. Bake
or grill until the cheese melts. Add in a large tossed
salad topped with your favorite fat free dressing.
Finish up with an apple or orange.

Afternoon snack:
Three cups air popped popcorn

Dinner:
Steak and salad
Cook a 4 ounce sirloin steak to your liking. Team
with 3 boiled new potatoes, ½ cup of white bean
salad (see p. 182 of our book *The Glucose
Revolution* for a recipe or just use a canned mixed
bean salad). Add a green salad, dressed with 1
tablespoon vinaigrette.

Evening snack:
A generous wedge of cantaloupe (about 2 cups)

Chapter 14

G.I. SUCCESS STORIES

*J*ust in case you're not yet convinced that a low G.I. diet can help you lose weight, dietitian Johanna Burani, M.S., R.D., C.D.E., offers these three real-life examples from her own practice. Many of Johanna's patients have lost weight, controlled their diabetes and gained overall better health by choosing a low G.I. way of life.

CASE STUDY #1
"Marge"

Age: 33
Height: 5'4¾"
Weight: 246 pounds (clinically defined as "morbidly obese")

Background:
Marge is a single mother who smokes one pack of cigarettes a day, drinks alcoholic beverages socially and does no deliberate exercise.

Marge's "before" diet:
Breakfast: Fried bacon and eggs, 2 slices white toast with butter, water

Lunch (which she skips once or twice a week): usually eats at a fast-food restaurant. Typical meal: Quarter-pounder with cheese, large French fries, diet Coke

Late afternoon snack: Handful of chocolate kisses, 5 or 6 Ritz crackers, Cheddar cheese

Dinner: Steak, baked potato with butter, small portion of broccoli, instant pudding

Late night snack: Large bowl of ice cream

MARGE'S "BEFORE" NUTRITIONAL ANALYSIS:

Calories: 3600
Carbohydrate: 185 g (21%)
Protein: 157 g (18%)
Fat: 246 g (61%)
G.I.: 74

Johanna's nutritional assessment:
To lose weight, Marge had to decrease her caloric intake, and specifically the amount of fat she was eating. To improve the nutrient balance of her meals and snacks, she would need to include at least 5 servings of fruits and vegetables, and 2 or 3 servings of dairy foods each day.

G.I.-specific counseling:

It was Marge's high fat intake that kept her feeling full. Grossly decreasing her dietary fat would leave her hungry, since her carbohydrate choices had high G.I. values.

By increasing her carbohydrate calories and selecting low G.I. foods, Marge could achieve the same sense of prolonged satiety (feelings of fullness) that fat provides, with fewer than half the calories!

Marge's new, low G.I. menu:

Breakfast: Two slices 100% stoneground whole wheat toast, 2 tablespoons natural peanut butter, 8 ozs. 1% milk and a handful of grapes

Snack: Six to 8 ozs. of light yogurt (plain or fruit flavored)

Lunch: Two-ounce pita, 2 ozs. roasted turkey breast, lettuce and tomato, large mixed salad with fat free dressing, an orange and decaf diet beverage

Dinner: Shrimp teriyaki stir fry: ⅔ cup Uncle Ben's Converted Rice, 4 ozs. shrimp, at least 1 cup Oriental vegetables (fresh or frozen), 3 ozs. cherries and herbal diet iced tea or water

Snack: Eight ozs. 1% milk and a large oatmeal cookie

MARGE'S "AFTER" NUTRITIONAL ANALYSIS:

Calories: 1600
Carbohydrate: 231 g (56%)
Protein: 93 g (23%)
Fat: 38 g (21%)
G.I.: 43

Marge's winning results:
Marge has been following her low G.I. meal plan for two and a half years. So far, she has lost 72 pounds (current weight: 174 pounds). Her goal weight is 160 pounds.

Marge's comments:
"I can't believe I'm never hungry. This is such an easy way to lose weight—and I don't consider this a diet. I love how I look and feel!"

CASE STUDY #2
"Annie"

Age: 7
Height: 3'8"
Weight: 80 pounds (clinically defined as "morbidly obese")

Background:
Annie is a second grader who lives at home with her parents and a younger sibling. No one else in her family has a weight problem. Annie's pediatrician advised Annie's mother to seek nutritional guidance from an R.D. to help her gradually lose approximately 10 pounds over the next year. Annie's mother admitted to a lack of nutritional knowledge, but emphasized the whole family's willingness to implement Johanna's recommended dietary changes.

Annie's "before" diet:
Breakfast: A ¾ oz. serving of Rice Chex and 4 ozs. 1% milk
Snack: An 8 oz. glass of milk and a breakfast bar
Lunch: Turkey breast on a small roll, ½ cup instant mashed potatoes with gravy and 8 ozs. 1% milk

Snack: Two Oreo cookies and an ice cream sandwich
Dinner: Small bowl of commercial chicken noodle soup with 5 saltines and a cup of orange soda
Late night snack: One-half orange

ANNIE'S "BEFORE" NUTRITIONAL ANALYSIS:

Calories: 1700
Carbohydrate: 251 g (60%)
Protein: 64 g (15%)
Fat: 46 g (25%)
G.I.: 70

Johanna's nutritional assessment:
Annie's diet contains multiple nutritional problems.

- Her morbid obesity at such a young age predisposes her to weight-related health problems later in life if she doesn't make changes now.
- While her milk consumption appears to meet at least the minimal calcium needs of a seven-year-old child, her other quality protein foods (meat, fish, eggs, and so on) may be lacking on some days.
- Her fiber intake is inadequate because she eats very little fruit, vegetables and whole grains; her consumption of vitamins and minerals is also likely to be inadequate.
- She complains of being too tired to play after school.
- She is hungry all the time.

G.I.-specific counseling:
By decreasing her excessive carbohydrate intake

(most of which are high G.I. foods), and substituting low G.I. fruits, vegetables and whole grains, Annie will start consuming fewer—yet still enough—calories, have more energy and feel fuller, longer. And in the process, Annie will enjoy a balanced meal plan to meet the demanding nutrient needs of a growing seven year old!

Annie's new, low G.I. menu:
Breakfast: Three-quarters cup Quaker Life cereal, 4 ozs. 1% milk and ½ banana
Snack: One-half sandwich bag of green grapes (about 17), 4 ozs. 1% milk
Lunch: A ham and Swiss sandwich on 2 slices rye bread with lettuce, tomato and mustard, 10 baby carrots, 4 ozs. 1% milk
Snack: Four Social Tea biscuits, 4 ozs. 1% milk
Dinner: Chicken leg, breaded without the skin, ½ cup mashed sweet potato, ½ cups green beans vinaigrette, ½ cup natural applesauce, 4 ozs. 1% milk
Snack: One-half cup low fat pudding

ANNIE'S "AFTER" NUTRITIONAL ANALYSIS:

Calories: 1400
Carbohydrate: 196 g (58%)
Protein: 74 g (22%)
Fat: 31 g (20%)
G.I.: 51

Annie's winning results:
Over the past eight months, Annie has lost 7 pounds and has grown an inch. Her weight is finally back on the height/weight growth chart again. Annie's doctor

wants her to continue her current dietary regimen and check back in six months.

Annie's comments:
Annie's mother is thrilled to see her little girl less moody with more energy. She is particularly happy that meal and snack times are no longer tumultuous battles.

CASE STUDY #3
"Bill"

Age: 43
Height: 5'10"
Weight: 245 pounds (clinically defined as "morbidly obese")

Background:
Bill works as a stock broker who commutes three hours to and from his office each day. For exercise, he bikes or walks for 30 to 45 minutes, three or four times a week. He doesn't drink much water and drinks alcohol on the weekends. Over the past two years, Bill has gained 35 pounds. Bill's diet revealed a huge disparity between what he eats on "good" and "bad" days: Below is one of Bill's "bad" days.

BILL'S "BEFORE" DIET:

Breakfast: Two slices of rye toast with jelly, 2 cups of coffee
Snack: A large cheese Danish and a cup of coffee
Lunch: A bowl of chicken soup, roast beef and provolone hoagie, cole slaw, large order of French fries, large cup of low fat frozen yogurt with M&M topping and 2 large glasses of sweetened iced tea

Dinner: Broiled chicken breast stuffed with spinach, large portion of eggplant parmesan, ½ large French baguette and wine

Late night snack: Ten peanut butter Girl Scout cookies with 16 ozs. of skim milk

---

BILL'S "BEFORE" NUTRITIONAL ANALYSIS:

Calories: 5500
Carbohydrate: 544 g (40%)
Protein: 244 g (18%)
Fat: 258 g (42%)
G.I.: 73

Johanna's nutritional assessment:
The only chance Bill has to lose weight is to reduce his calorie intake to a reasonable level and to eat a consistent number of calories from day to day. By varying his food consumption so drastically (from 1,300 calories on "good" days to more than 5,000 on "bad" days), he was actually programming his body to store more fat!

G.I.-specific counseling:
Because his days are long, Bill needs nutrient-dense, sustaining meals and snacks. Replacing nearly 75 percent of his excessive fat calories with low G.I. foods would give him the satiety he was accustomed to for a small fraction of the calories.

Bill's new, low G.I. menu:
Breakfast: One and one-third cups Fiber One cereal, 8 ozs. of skim milk and 1 whole grapefruit
Lunch: A roast beef sandwich with lettuce and toma-

to in a large pita, large tossed salad with fat free
dressing, 8 ozs. skim milk
Snack: A 1½ cup portion of fresh fruit salad
Dinner: One cup steamed brown rice, 4 ozs. pork
tenderloin (roasted), 1 cup spinach with garlic and
olive oil, tossed salad (if desired), water or small glass
of wine, 4 ozs. natural applesauce
Snack: Three graham crackers, 8 ozs. skim milk

BILL'S "AFTER" NUTRITIONAL ANALYSIS:

Calories: 2000
Carbohydrate: 251 g (50%)
Protein: 112 g (22%)
Fat: 62 g (28%)
G.I.: 47

Bill's winning results:
In nine months, Bill has lost 45 pounds, bringing him
to his goal weight of 200 pounds. Four years later, he
is happily maintaining his goal weight!

Bill's comments:
"I like the foods I'm eating. The best part, though, is
that I'm not so draggy when I get home at night. I
still have energy to enjoy my family."

Chapter 15

YOUR QUESTIONS ANSWERED

WHICH IS BETTER FOR WEIGHT LOSS:
HIGH PROTEIN OR LOW G.I. FOODS?

CAN I EAT ALL THE CARBOHYDRATE I WANT
AND STILL LOSE WEIGHT?

HOW CAN I AVOID HUNGER PANGS?

AREN'T POTATOES AND BREAD FATTENING?

AND MORE . . .

Why are diets that disregard widely accepted nutritional guidelines so fashionable right now?

Several best-selling books have been published promoting high protein diets and generating a lot of publicity. They have been seized upon as a viable weight loss panacea. But the fact is: Diets that limit major food groups do not work over the long haul.

What are the side effects of a high protein diet?

The body cannot process large quantities of protein, so excess waste is produced that can overburden the kidneys. Not only can some high protein diets make existing kidney problems worse, but they also can cause mild renal failure to progress faster. Some high protein diets are also harmful for elderly people and anyone with high blood pressure or diabetes. High protein, high fat diets can lead to high cholesterol, heart disease, and increase the risk of heart attack. Further, some high protein diets reduce the intake of important vitamins, minerals, fiber and trace elements. They also lack fiber, which may lead to constipation.

Why do people on high protein diets shed pounds?

Because they make people lose water weight. Overweight people need to lose body fat—not muscle or water. And the way to do this is by eating a balanced diet of low glycemic index carbohydrates and burning more calories than we take in.

How do high carbohydrate, low G.I. diets help people to lose weight?

- Because low G.I. diets lower insulin levels, over the long term you'll burn more—and store less—fat. (Insulin determines how much fat we store and burn.)
- You're less likely to overeat low G.I. carbohydrates, because they're bulky and filling. Consider them natural appetite suppressants!
- A low G.I. diet offers you plenty of food choices, so you're less likely to feel deprived. Unlike diets that restrict certain foods, a low G.I. diet is easy to live with.

Can I still lose weight eating as much carbohydrate as I want?

Possibly not. We recommend a high carbohydrate intake and a low fat intake. While carbohydrate is not usually stored as fat, if you are eating more total energy than your body requires, then the carbohydrate will be used as a source of fuel in preference to fat. This would have the effect of limiting the break-down of body fat stores. The idea is to eat enough energy in total to satisfy your appetite (using low G.I. foods helps) and nutritional requirements, but not more than you need. An increase in your activity level will help burn up body fat as it is used as an additional fuel.

I've always heard that sugar is fattening. Is it?

No. Sugar has no special fattening properties—in fact, it is no more likely to be turned into fat than any other carbohydrate. Sugar, which you'll often find in foods high in calories and fat may sometimes seem to be "turned into fat," but it's the total number of calories you're consuming rather than the sugar in those calorie dense foods that may contribute to new stores of fat.

What is chana dal?

Chana dal, the bean with the lowest glycemic index (G.I. 8), is a diet staple in India, but, as yet, is still little known in the United States. Scientifically, chana dal is the *desi* type of *Cicer arietinum*. The chana dal bean looks just like yellow split peas, but when cooked, it doesn't readily boil down to mush the way split peas do. It is more closely related to chickpeas (garbanzo beans), but chana dal is younger, smaller, sweeter, and has a much lower glycemic index. In fact, you can substitute chana dal for chickpeas in just about any recipe. Chana dal is generally available in Indian and Southeast Asian food stores, and as awareness of the value of eating low G.I. foods spreads, it is becoming more widely available. If you don't see it at your favorite food store, ask your local health food store or specialty grocer to carry it.

What effect does fiber have on the G.I. value?

There is no simple answer to this question. Dietary fiber is not one chemical constituent, as fat and protein are. It is composed of many different sorts of molecules. Fiber can lower the glycemic index in some foods and not in others, depending on its physical form.

Soluble fiber tends to be viscous (thick and jellylike) and can slow down digestion. Thus, the presence of soluble fiber in such foods as oats and legumes may contribute to their low glycemic index values. Purified psyllium added to foods slows down digestion because it is also viscous.

Insoluble fiber in flours is finely ground and often doesn't slow digestion. Whole wheat bread and white bread have similar glycemic index values. Brown pasta and brown rice have similar values to their white counterparts. Sometimes insoluble fiber acts as a physical barrier that prevents the enzymes from attacking the starch. Whole (intact) grains of wheat, rye and barley have lower glycemic index values than cracked grains.

Chapter 16

CUTTING THE FAT: YOUR A TO Z GUIDE

As we have said constantly throughout this book, it is important to eat a high carbohydrate and low fat diet. The following practical tips that we have set out in an easy A to Z format will help you reduce the fat content of some of your favorite recipes while lowering their glycemic index.

Alcohol
Although excessive alcohol consumption can be fattening, as an ingredient in a recipe, alcohol itself won't create a high calorie dish. Alcohol evaporates during cooking, so you lose the calories and are left with the flavor. A little wine in a sauce can give a delicious flavor, and sherry in an Asian style marinade is essential.

Bacon

Bacon is a valuable ingredient in many dishes because of the flavor it offers. You can make a little bacon go a long way by trimming off all fat and chopping it finely. Lean ham is often a more economical and leaner way to go. In casseroles and soups, a ham bone imparts a fine flavor without much fat.

Cheese

At around 30 percent fat (23 percent of it saturated), cheese can contribute quite a lot of fat to a recipe. Although there are a number of fat-reduced cheeses available, many of these lose a lot in flavor for a small reduction in fat. It is worth comparing fat per ounce between brands to find the tastiest one with the lowest fat content. Alternatively, a sprinkle of a grated, very tasty cheese or Parmesan may do the job.

Part skim ricotta and cottage cheeses are lower fat alternatives to butter on a sandwich. It's worth trying some fresh part skim ricotta from a deli—you may find the texture and flavor more acceptable than that of the ricotta available in containers in the supermarket. Flavored cottage cheeses are ideal low fat toppings for crackers. Try ricotta in lasagna instead of a creamy white sauce.

Cream and sour cream

Keep to very small amounts as these are high in saturated fat. Substitute nonfat sour cream, which tastes very similar to the full fat variety. A 16 ounce container of heavy cream can be poured into ice-cube trays and frozen providing small servings of cream easily when you need it. Adding one ice-cube block (1 oz.) of cream to a dish adds only 5½ grams of fat.

Dried beans, peas and lentils

These are all low in fat and very nutritious. Incorporating them in a recipe, perhaps as partial substitution of meat, will lower the fat content of the finished product. Canned beans, chickpeas and lentils are now widely available. They are very convenient to use and a great time saver. They are comparable in food value to the dried ones that you soak and cook yourself.

Eggs

Be conscious of eggs in a recipe as they can add fat. Sometimes just the beaten egg white can be substituted for the whole egg, or use real egg substitute.

Filo Pastry

Unlike most other pastry, filo (also known as phyllo) is low in fat. To keep it that way, brush between the sheets with skim milk instead of melted butter when you prepare it. Look for it in the freezer section of the supermarket with other prepared pastry and use it as a pie filling or a strudel wrap.

Grilling

Grill or broil tender cuts of meat, chicken and fish rather than fry. Marinating first will add flavor, moisture and tenderness. Grilling vegetables is a great way to bring out their utmost flavor.

Health food stores

Health food stores can be traps for the unwary. Check out the high fat ingredients, such as hydrogenated vegetable oil, nuts, coconut and palm kernel oil in the products such as granola bars, fruit bars and "healthy" cakes (even if made with whole wheat flour) that they stock on their shelves.

Ice cream
A source of carbohydrate, calcium, riboflavin, retinol and protein and low fat varieties have lower glycemic index values—definitely a nutritious and icy treat.

Jam
A tablespoon of jam on toast contains far fewer calories than a pat of butter. So, enjoy your jam and give fat the flick!

Keep jars of minced garlic, chili or ginger in the refrigerator to pice up your cooking in an instant.

Lemon juice
Try a fresh squeeze with ground black pepper on vegetables rather than a pat of butter. Lemon juice provides acidity that slows gastric emptying and lowers the glycemic index.

Milk
Many people dislike skim milk, particularly when they taste it on its own or in their coffee! However, you can use skim milk in a recipe and no one will notice—and the fat savings is great. For convenience you might want to keep powdered skim milk in the pantry, which can be made up to the desired quantity when you need it. It will taste more like fresh milk if you mix the powder and water according to directions and refrigerate the milk overnight before using it. Ultra-pasteurized (or shelf stable) milk is handy in the cupboard, too.

Nuts
They are valuable for their content of vitamin E, but they are also high in fat. To keep the fat content of a recipe low, the quantity of nuts has to be small.

Oil

Most of our recipes call for no more than 2 tea-spoons of oil. Any polyunsaturated or monounsaturated oil is suitable. Cooking spray or brushing oil lightly over the base of the pan is ideal. If you find the amount of oil insufficient, cover your pan, or add a few drops of water and use steam to cook the ingredients without burning. It is a good idea to invest in a nonstick frying pan if you don't have one!

Pasta

A food to eat more of and a great source of carbohydrate and B vitamins. Fresh or dried, the preparation is easy. Just boil in water until just tender or "al dente," drain and top with a dollop of pesto, a tomato sauce or a sprinkle of Parmesan and pepper. There are many wonderful pasta cookbooks now available, and it's definitely worth investing in one to find all sorts of exciting ways to prepare this fabulous low G.I. food. Pasta may appear in your menu as a side dish to meat, as noodles in soup, as a meal in itself with vegetables or sauce or even as an ingredient in a dessert.

Questions

Ask your dietitian for more recipe ideas. (See page 110 in "For More Information" for guidance on finding a dietitian near you.)

Reduce the fat content of ground beef by browning it in a nonstick pan, then placing the meat in a colander and pouring boiling water through it to wash away the fat. Return to the pan to continue cooking. It is a good idea to buy the better quality ground beef with less fat.

Stock

If you are prepared to go to the effort of making your own stock—good for you! Prepare it in advance, refrigerate it then skim off the accumulated fat from the top. Prepared stock is available in long-life cartons and cans in the supermarket. Stock cubes are another alternative. Look for brands that have reduced salt.

To sauté

Heat the pan first, brush with the recommended amount of oil (or less), add the food and cook, stirring lightly over a gentle heat.

Underlying the need for fat is a need for taste. Be creative with other flavorings.

Vinegar

A vinaigrette dressing (1 tablespoon vinegar and 2 teaspoons of oil) with your salad can lower the blood sugar response to the whole meal by up to 30 percent. The best types of vinegars for this purpose are red or white wine vinegar, or use lemon juice.

Weighing

What's the weight of the meat you're buying? Start noticing the weight that appears on the butcher's scales or package label and consider how many servings it will give you. With a food such as steak, that is basically all edible meat, 4 to 5 ounces per serving is sufficient. One pound is more than enough for 4 portions. Choose lean cuts of meat and trim away the fat before cooking or before you put it away. Alternate meat or chicken with fish once or twice a week.

Yogurt

Yogurt is a valuable food in many ways. It is a good source of calcium, "friendly bacteria," protein and riboflavin, and unlike milk, is suitable for those people who are lactose intolerant. Low fat plain yogurt is a suitable substitute for sour cream. If using yogurt in a hot sauce or casserole, add it at the last minute and do not let it boil, or it will curdle. It is best if you can bring the yogurt to room temperature before adding to the hot dish. To do this, mix a small amount of yogurt with a little sauce from the dish, then stir this mixture back into the bulk of the sauce.

Zero fat

Eating zero fat is unhealthy, so speak with a dietitian about how to get just the right amount you need. Our bodies need essential fatty acids that can't be synthesized and must be supplied in the diet. Fat does add flavor—use it to your advantage.

Chapter 17

HOW TO USE THE G.I. TABLE

*T*he following table is an A to Z listing of the glycemic index of commonly eaten foods in the United States and Canada. Approximately 300 different foods are listed, including some new values for foods tested only recently.

The G.I. value shown next to each food is the average for that food using glucose as the standard (i.e., glucose has a G.I. value of 100, with other foods rated accordingly). The average may represent the mean of 10 studies of that food worldwide or only 2 to 4 studies. In a few instances, American data are different from the rest of the world and we show that data rather than the average. Rice and oatmeal fall into this category.

To check on a food's glycemic index, simply look

for it by name in the alphabetic list. You may also find it under a food type, as fruit or cookies, for example.

Included in the tables is the carbohydrate (CHO) and fat content of a sample serving of the food. This is to help you keep track of the amount of fat and carbohydrate in your diet. The sample serving is not the recommended serving—it is just an example of a serving. The glycemic index does not depend on your serving size because it is a ranking of the glycemic effect of foods using carbohydrate-equivalent portion sizes. You can eat more of a low G.I. food or less of a high G.I. food and achieve the same blood sugar levels.

Remember when you are choosing foods, the glycemic index isn't the only thing to consider. In terms of your blood sugar levels you should also consider the amount of carbohydrate you are eating. For your overall health the fat, fiber and micronutrient content of your diet is also important. A dietitian can guide you further with good food choices; see "For More Information" on page 110 for advice on finding a dietitian.

■

FOR A SMALL EATER (1,500 CALORIES A DAY),
AIM FOR LESS THAN 50 G FAT A DAY
AND 188 G CARBOHYDRATE.

■

FOR A BIGGER EATER (2,500 CALORIES A DAY),
AIM FOR LESS THAN 80 G FAT A DAY
AND 313 G CARBOHYDRATE.

■

Chapter 18

THE GLYCEMIC INDEX TABLE

A–Z OF FOODS WITH GLYCEMIC INDEX, CARBOHYDRATE & FAT

Food	Glycemic Index	Fat (g per svg.)	CHO (g per svg.)
Agave nectar (90% fructose syrup), 1 tablespoon	11	0	16
All-Bran with extra fiber™, Kellogg's, breakfast cereal, ½ cup, 1 oz.	51 (av)	1	22
Angel food cake, ½₂ cake, 1 oz.	67	trace	17
Apple, 1 medium, 5 ozs.	38 (av)	0	18
Apple, dried, 1 oz.	29	0	24
Apple juice, unsweetened, 1 cup, 8 ozs.	40	0	29
Apple cinnamon muffin, from mix, 1 muffin	44	5	26
Apricots, fresh, 3 medium, 3 ozs.	57	0	12
canned, light syrup, 3 halves	64	0	14
dried, 5 halves	31	0	13
Apricot jam, no added sugar, 1 tablespoon	55	0	17
Apricot and honey muffin, low fat, from mix, 1 muffin	60	4	27
Bagel, 1 small, plain, 2.3 ozs.	72	1	38
Baked beans, ½ cup, 4 ozs.	48 (av)	1	24
Banana bread, 1 slice, 3 ozs.	47	7	46
Banana, raw, 1 medium, 5 ozs.	55 (av)	0	32
Banana, oat and honey muffin, low fat from mix, 1 muffin	65	4	27
Barley, pearled, boiled, ½ cup, 2.6 ozs.	25 (av)	0	22
Basmati white rice, boiled, 1 cup, 6 ozs.	58	0	50
Beets, canned, drained, ½ cup, 3 ozs.	64	0	5
Black bean soup, ½ cup, 4 ½ ozs.	64	2	19
Black beans, boiled, ¾ cup, 4.3 ozs.	30	1	31
Black bread, dark rye, 1 slice, 1.7 ozs.	76	1	18
Blackeyed peas, canned, ½ cup, 4 ozs.	42	1	16
Blueberry muffin, 1 muffin, 2 ozs.	59	4	27
Bran			
All-Bran with extra fiber™, Kellogg's, ½ cup, 1 oz.	51	1	20

Food	Glycemic Index	Fat (g per svg.)	CHO (g per svg.)
Bran Buds with Psyllium™, Kellogg's, ⅓ cup, 1 oz.	45	1	24
Bran Flakes, Post, ⅔ cup, 1 oz.	74	1	22
Multi-Bran Chex™, General Mills, 1 cup, 2.1 ozs.	58	15	49
Oat bran, 1 tablespoon	55	1	7
Oat bran muffin, 2 ozs.	60	4	28
Rice bran, 1 tablespoon	19	2	5
Breads			
Dark rye, Black bread, 1 slice, 1.7 ozs.	76	1	18
Dark rye, Schinkenbröt, 1 slice, 2 ozs.	86	1	22
French baguette, 1 oz.	95	1	15
Gluten-free bread, 1 slice	90	1	18
Hamburger bun, 1 prepacked bun, 1½ ozs.	61	2	22
Kaiser roll, 1, 2 ozs.	73	2	34
Light deli (American) rye, 1 slice, 1 oz.	68	1	16
Melba toast, 6 pieces, 1 oz.	70	2	23
Natural Ovens 100% Whole Grain, 1 slice, 1.2 ozs.	51	0	17
Natural Ovens Hunger Filler, 1 slice, 1.2 ozs.	59	0	16
Natural Ovens Natural Wheat, 1 slice, 1.2 ozs.	59	0	16
Natural Ovens Happiness, 1 slice, 1.1 oz.	63	0	15
Pita bread, whole wheat, 6½ inch loaf, 2 ozs.	57	2	35
Pumpernickel, whole grain, 1 slice, 1 oz.	51	1	15
Rye bread, 1 slice, 1 oz.	65	1	15
Sourdough, 1 slice, 1½ ozs.	52	1	20
Sourdough rye, Arnold's, 1 slice, 1½ ozs.	57	1	21
White, 1 slice, 1 oz.	70 (av)	1	12
100% stoneground whole wheat, 1 slice, 1½ ozs.	53	1	15
Whole wheat, 1 slice, 1 oz.	69 (av)	1	13
Bread stuffing from mix, 2 ozs.	74	5	13
Breakfast cereals			
All-Bran with extra fiber™, Kellogg's, ½ cup, 1 oz.	51	1	20
Bran Buds with Psyllium™, Kellogg's, ½ cup, 1 oz.	45	1	24
Bran Flakes, Post, ⅔ cup, 1 oz.	74	1	22
Cheerios™, General Mills, 1 cup, 1 oz.	74	2	23
Cocoa Krispies™, Kellogg's, 1 cup, 1 oz.	77	1	27
Corn Bran™, Quaker Crunchy, ¾ cup, 1 oz.	75	1	23
Corn Chex™, Nabisco, 1 cup, 1 oz.	83	0	26
Corn Flakes™, Kellogg's, 1 cup, 1 oz.	84 (av)	0	24
Cream of Wheat, instant, 1 packet, 1 oz.	74	0	21

Food	Glycemic Index	Fat (g per svg.)	CHO (g per svg.)
Cream of Wheat, old fashioned, ¾ cup, cooked, 6 ozs.	66	0	21
Crispix™, Kellogg's, 1 cup, 1 oz.	87	0	25
Frosted Flakes™, Kellogg's, ¾ cup, 1 oz.	55	0	28
Golden Grahams™, General Mills, ¾ cup, 1.6 ozs.	71	1	25
Grapenuts™, Post, ¼ cup, 1 oz.	67	1	27
Grapenuts Flakes™, Post, ¾ cup, 1 oz.	80	1	24
Life™, Quaker, ¾ cup, 1 oz.	66	1	25
Muesli, natural muesli, ⅔ cup, 1½ ozs.	56	3	28
Muesli, toasted, ⅔ cup, 2 ozs.	43	10	41
Multi-Bran Chex™, General Mills, 1 cup, 2.1 ozs.	58	1.5	49
Oat bran, raw, 1 tablespoon	55	1	7
Oat bran™, Quaker Oats, ¾ cup, 1 oz.	50	1	23
Oatmeal (made with water), old fashioned, cooked, ½ cup, 4 ozs.	49 (av)	1	12
Oats, 1-minute, Quaker Oats, 1 cup, cooked	66	2	25
Puffed Wheat™, Quaker, 2 cups, 1 oz.	67	0	22
Raisin Bran™, Kellogg's, ¾ cup, 1 oz.	73	0	32
Rice bran, 1 tablespoon	19	2	5
Rice Chex™, General Mills, 1¼ cups, 1 oz.	89	0	27
Rice Krispies™, Kellogg's, 1¼ cups, 1 oz.	82	0	26
Shredded wheat, spoonsize, ⅔ cup, 1.2 ozs.	58	0	27
Shredded Wheat™, Post, 1 oz.	83	1	23
Smacks™, Kellogg's, ¾ cup, 1 oz.	56	1	24
Special K™, Kellogg's, 1 cup, 1 oz.	66	0	22
Team Flakes™, Nabisco, ¾ cup, 1 oz.	82	0	25
Total™, General Mills, ¾ cup, 1 oz.	76	1	24
Weetabix™, 2 biscuits, 1.2 ozs.	75	1	28
Buckwheat groats, cooked, ½ cup, 2.7 ozs.	54 (av)	1	20
Bulgur, cooked, ⅔ cup, 4 ozs.	48 (av)	0	23
Bun, hamburger, 1 prepacked bun, 1.7 ozs.	61	2	22
Butter beans, boiled, ½ cup, 4 ozs.	31 (av)	0	16
Cakes			
Angel food cake, 1 slice, 1/12 cake, 1 oz.	67	trace	17
Banana bread, 1 slice, 3 ozs.	47	7	46
Pound cake, homemade, 1 slice, 3 ozs.	54	15	42
Sponge cake, 1 slice, 1/12 cake, 2 ozs.	46	4	32
Capellini pasta, cooked, 1 cup, 6 ozs.	45	1	53

Food	Glycemic Index	Fat (g per svg.)	CHO (g per svg.)
Cantaloupe, raw, ¼ small, 6½ ozs.	65	0	16
Carrots, peeled, boiled, canned, ½ cup, 2.4 ozs.	49	0	3
Carrots, peeled, boiled, canned, ½ cup, 2.4 ozs.	49	0	3
Cereal grains			
Barley, pearled, boiled, ½ cup, 2.6 ozs.	25 (av)	0	22
Bulgur, cooked, ½ cup, 3 ozs.	48 (av)	0	17
Couscous, cooked, ½ cup, 3 ozs.	65 (av)	0	21
Corn			
Cornmeal, whole grain, from mix, cooked, ⅓ cup, 1.4 ozs.	68	1	30
Sweet corn, canned, drained, ½ cup, 3 ozs.	55 (av)	1	15
Taco shells, 2 shells, 1 oz.	68	5	17
Rice			
Basmati, white, boiled, 1 cup, 6 ozs.	58	0	50
Brown, 1 cup, 6 ozs.	55 (av)	0	37
Converted™, Uncle Ben's, 1 cup, 6 ozs.	44	0	38
Instant, cooked, 1 cup, 6 ozs.	87	0	37
Long grain, white, 1 cup, 6 ozs.	56 (av)	0	42
Parboiled, 1 cup, 6 ozs.	48	0	38
Rice cakes, plain, 3 cakes, 1 oz.	82	1	23
Short grain, white, 1 cup, 6 ozs.	72	0	42
Chana dal, ½ cup, 4 ozs.	8	3	28
Cheerios™, General Mills, breakfast cereal, 1 cup, 1 oz.	74	2	23
Cherries, 10 large cherries, 3 ozs.	22	0	10
Chickpeas (garbanzo beans),canned, drained, ½ cup, 4 ozs.	42	2	15
boiled, ½ cup, 3 ozs.	33 (av)	2	23
Chocolate butterscotch muffin, low fat from mix, 1 muffin	53	4	29
Chocolate, bar, 1½ ozs.	49	14	26
Chocolate Flavor, Nestle Qulk™ (made with water), 3 teaspoons	53	0	14
Coca-Cola™, soft drink, 1 can	63	0	39
Cocoa Krispies™, Kellogg's, breakfast cereal, 1 cup, 1 oz.	77	1	27
Corn			
Cornmeal, cooked from mix, ⅓ cup, 1.4 ozs.	68	1	30
Sweet corn, canned and drained, ½ cup, 3 ozs.	55 (av)	1	15
Corn Bran™, Quaker Crunchy, breakfast cereal, ¾ cup, 1 oz.	75	1	23
Corn Chex™, General Mills, breakfast cereal, 1 cup, 1 oz.	83	0	26
Corn chips, 1 oz.	72	10	16
Corn Flakes™, Kellogg's, breakfast cereal, 1 cup, 1 oz.	84 (av)	0	24

Food	Glycemic Index	Fat (g per svg.)	CHO (g per svg.)
Cornmeal, from mix, cooked, ½ cup, 1.4 ozs.	68	1	30
Cookies			
Graham crackers, 4 squares, 1 oz.	74	3	22
Milk Arrowroot, 3 cookies, ½ oz.	69	2	9
Oatmeal, 1 cookie, ⅔ oz.	55	3	12
Shortbread, 4 small cookies, 1 oz.	64	7	19
Social Tea™ biscuits, Nabisco, 4 cookies, ⅔ oz.	55	3	13
Vanilla wafers, 7 cookies, 1 oz.	77	4	21
see also Crackers			
Couscous, cooked, ⅔ cup, 4 ozs.	65 (av)	0	21
Crackers			
Crispbread, 3 crackers, ⅔ oz.	81	0	15
Kavli™ All Natural Whole Grain Crispbread, 4 wafers, 1 oz.	71	1	16
Premium soda crackers, saltine, 8 crackers, 1 oz.	74	3	17
Rice cakes, plain, 3 cakes, 1 oz.	82	1	23
Ryvita™ Tasty Dark Rye Whole Grain Crisp Bread, 2 slices, ⅔ oz.	69	1	16
Stoned wheat thins, 3 crackers, ⅓ oz.	67	2	15
Water cracker, Carr's, 3 king size crackers, ⅔ oz.	78	2	18
Cream of Wheat, instant, 1 packet, 1 oz.	74	0	21
Cream of Wheat, old fashioned, ¾ cup, cooked, 6 ozs.	66	0	21
Crispix™, Kellogg's, breakfast cereal, 1 cup, 1 oz.	87	0	25
Croissant, medium, 1.2 ozs.	67	14	27
Custard, ½ cup, 4.4 ozs.	43	4	24
Dairy foods and nondairy substitutes			
Ice cream, 10% fat, vanilla, ½ cup, 2.2 ozs.	61 (av)	7	16
Ice milk, vanilla, ½ cup, 2.2 ozs.	50	3	15
Milk, whole, 1 cup, 8 ozs.	27 (av)	9	11
skim, 1 cup, 8 ozs.	32	0	12
chocolate flavored, 1%, 1 cup, 8 ozs.	34	3	26
Pudding, ½ cup, 4.4 ozs.	43	4	24
Soy milk, 1 cup, 8 ozs.	31	7	14
Tofu frozen dessert (nondairy), low fat, ½ cup, 2 ozs.	115	1	21
Yogurt			
nonfat, fruit flavored, with sugar, 8 ozs.	33	0	30
nonfat, plain, artificial sweetener, 8 ozs.	14	0	17
nonfat, fruit flavored, artificial sweetener, 8 ozs.	14	0	16
Dates, dried, 5, 1.4 ozs.	103	0	27

Food	Glycemic Index	Fat (g per svg.)	CHO (g per svg.)
Doughnut with cinnamon and sugar, 1.6 ozs.	76	11	29
Fanta™, soft drink, 1 can	68	0	47
Fava beans, frozen, boiled, ½ cup, 3 ozs.	79	0	17
Fettucine, cooked, 1 cup, 6 ozs.	32	1	57
Fish sticks, frozen, oven-cooked, fingers, 3½ ozs.	38	14	24
Flan cake, ½ cup, 4 ozs.	65	5	23
French baguette bread, 1 oz.	95	0	15
French fries, large, 4.3 ozs.	75	22	46
Frosted Flakes™, Kellogg's, breakfast cereal, ¾ cup, 1 oz.	55	0	28
Fructose, pure, 3 packets	23 (av)	0	10
Fruit cocktail, canned in natural juice, ½ cup, 4 ozs.	55	0	15
Fruits and fruit products			
Agave nectar (90% fructose syrup), 1 tablespoon	11	0	16
Apple, 1 medium, 5 ozs.	38 (av)	0	18
Apple, dried, 1 oz.	29	0	24
Apple juice, unsweetened, 1 cup, 8 ozs.	40	0	29
Apricots, fresh, 3 medium, 3.3 ozs.	57	0	12
canned, light syrup, 3 halves	64	0	19
dried, 1 oz.	31	0	13
Apricot jam, no added sugar, 1 tablespoon	55	0	17
Banana, raw, 1 medium, 5 ozs.	55 (av)	0	32
Cantaloupe, raw, ¼ small, 6½ ozs.	65	0	16
Cherries, 10 large, 3 ozs.	22	0	10
Dates, dried, 5, 1.4 ozs.	103	0	27
Fruit cocktail, canned in natural juice, ½ cup, 4 ozs.	55	0	15
Grapefruit, raw, ½ medium, 3.3 ozs.	25	0	5
Grapefruit juice, unsweetened, 1 cup, 8 ozs.	48	0	22
Grapes, green, 1 cup, 3 ozs.	46 (av)	0	15
Kiwi, 1 medium, raw, peeled, 2½ ozs.	52 (av)	0	8
Mango, 1 small, 5 ozs.	55 (av)	0	19
Marmalade, 1 tablespoon	48	0	17
Orange, navel, 1 medium, 4 ozs.	44 (av)	0	10
Orange juice, 1 cup, 8 ozs.	46	0	26
Papaya, ½ medium, 5 ozs.	58 (av)	0	14
Peach, fresh, 1 medium, 3 ozs.	28	0	7
canned, natural juice, ½ cup, 4 ozs.	30	0	14
canned, light syrup, ½ cup, 4 ozs.	52	0	18
canned, heavy syrup, ½ cup, 4 ozs.	58	0	26

Food	Glycemic Index	Fat (g per svg.)	CHO (g per svg.)
Pear, fresh, 1 medium, 5 ozs.	38 (av)	0	21
canned in pear juice, ½ cup, 4 ozs.	44	0	13
Pineapple, fresh, 2 slices, 4 ozs.	66	0	10
Pineapple juice, unsweetened, canned, 8 ozs.	46	0	34
Plums, 1 medium, 2 ozs.	39 (av)	0	7
Raisins, ¼ cup, 1 oz.	64	0	28
Strawberry jam, 1 tablespoon	51	0	18
Watermelon, 1 cup, 5 ozs.	72	0	8
Gatorade™ sports drink, 1 cup, 8 ozs.	78	0	14
Glucose powder, 2½ tablets	102	0	10
Gluten-free bread, 1 slice, 1 oz.	90	1	18
Golden Grahams™, General Mills, ¾ cup, 1.6 ozs.	71	1	25
Granola Bars™, Quaker Chewy, 1 oz.	61	2	23
Gnocchi, cooked, 1 cup, 5 ozs.	68	3	71
Graham crackers, 4 squares, 1 oz.	74	3	22
Grapefruit, raw, ½ medium, 3.3 ozs.	25	0	5
Grapefruit juice unsweetened, 1 cup, 8 ozs.	48	0	22
Grapenuts™, Post, breakfast cereal, ¼ cup, 1 oz.	67	1	27
Grapenuts Flakes™, Post, breakfast cereal, ¾ cup, 1 oz.	80	1	24
Grapes, green, 1 cup, 3.3 ozs.	46 (av)	0	15
Green pea soup, canned, ready to serve, 1 cup, 9 ozs.	66	3	27
Hamburger bun, 1 prepacked bun, 1½ ozs.	61	2	22
Honey, 1 tablespoon	58	0	16
Ice cream, 10% fat, vanilla, ½ cup, 2.2 ozs.	61 (av)	7	16
Ice milk, vanilla, ½ cup, 2.2 ozs.	50	3	15
Isostar, 1 cup, 8 ozs.	73	0	18
Jelly beans, 10 large, 1 oz.	80	0	26
Kaiser rolls, 1 roll, 2 ozs.	73	2	34
Kavli™ All Natural Whole Grain Crispbread, 4 wafers, 1 oz.	71	1	16
Kidney beans, red, boiled, ½ cup, 3 ozs.	27 (av)	0	20
Kidney beans, red, canned and drained, ½ cup, 4.3 ozs.	52	0	19
Kiwi, 1 medium, raw, peeled, 2½ ozs.	52 (av)	0	8
Kudos Granola Bars™ (whole grain), 1 bar, 1 oz.	62	5	20
Lactose, pure, .7 oz.	46 (av)	0	10
Lentil soup, Unico, canned, 1 cup, 8 ozs.	44	1	24
Lentils, green and brown, boiled, ½ cup, 3 ozs.	30 (av)	0	16
Lentils, red, boiled, 1.4 cup, 4 ozs.	26 (av)	0	27
Life™, Quaker, breakfast cereal, ¾ cup, 1 oz.	66	1	25

Food	Glycemic Index	Fat (g per svg.)	CHO (g per svg.)
Life Savers™, roll candy, 6 pieces, peppermint	70	0	10
Light deli (American) rye bread, 1 slice, 1 oz.	68	1	16
Lima beans, baby, frozen, ½ cup, 3 ozs.	32	0	17
Linguine pasta, thick, cooked, 1 cup, 6 ozs.	46 (av)	1	56
Linguine pasta, thin, cooked, 1 cup, 6 ozs.	55 (av)	1	56
M&M's Chocolate Candies Peanut™, 1.7 oz. package	33	13	30
Macaroni and Cheese Dinner™, Kraft packaged, cooked, 1 cup, 7 ozs.	64	17	48
Macaroni, cooked, 1 cup, 6 ozs.	45	1	52
Maltose (maltodextrin), pure, 2½ teaspoons	105	0	10
Mango, 1 small, 5 ozs.	55 (av)	0	19
Marmalade, 1 tablespoon	48	0	17
Mars Almond Bar™, 1.8 ozs.	65	12	31
Melba toast, 6 pieces, 1 oz.	70	2	23
Milk, whole, 1 cup, 8 ozs.	27 (av)	9	11
skim, 1 cup, 8 ozs.	32	0	12
chocolate flavored, 1%, 1 cup, 8 ozs.	34	3	26
Milk Arrowroot, 3 cookies, ½ oz.	63	2	9
Millet, cooked, ½ cup, 4 ozs.	71	1	2
Muesli, breakfast cereal, toasted, ⅔ cup, 2 ozs.	43	10	41
Muesli, non-toasted, ⅔ cup, 1½ ozs.	56	3	28
Multi-Bran Chex™, General Mills, 1 cup, 2.1 ozs.	58	1.5	49
Muffins			
Apple cinnamon, from mix, 1 muffin, 2 ozs.	44	8	33
Apricot and honey, low fat, from mix, 1 muffin	60	4	27
Banana, oat and honey, low fat, from mix, 1 muffin	65	4	27
Blueberry, 1 muffin, 2 ozs.	59	4	27
Chocolate butterscotch, low fat, from mix, 1 muffin	53	4	29
Oat and raisin, low fat, from mix, 1 muffin	54	3	28
Oat bran, 1 muffin, 2 ozs.	60	4	28
Mung beans, boiled, ½ cup, 3½ ozs.	38	1	18
Natural Ovens 100% Whole Grain bread, 1 slice, 1.2 ozs.	51	0	17
Natural Ovens Hunger Filler bread, 1 slice, 1.2 ozs.	59	0	16
Natural Ovens Natural Wheat bread, 1 slice, 1.2 ozs.	59	0	16
Natural Ovens Happiness bread, 1 slice, 1.1 ozs.	63	0	15
Navy beans, boiled, ½ cup, 3 ozs.	38 (av)	0	
Nutella™ (spread), 2 tablespoons, 1 oz.	33	9	19
Oat and raisin muffin, low fat from mix, 1 muffin	54	3	28

Food	Glycemic Index	Fat (g per svg.)	CHO (g per svg.)
Oat bran, 1 tablespoon	55	1	7
Oat bran™, Quaker Oats, breakfast cereal, ¾ cup, 1 oz.	50	1	23
Oat bran, 1 muffin, 2 ozs.	60	4	28
Oatmeal (made with water), old fashioned, cooked, 1 cup, 8 ozs.	49	2	26
Oatmeal cookie, 1, ⅔ oz.	55	3	12
Oats, 1-minute, Quaker Oats, 1 cup, cooked	66	2	25
Orange, navel, 1 medium, 4 ozs.	44 (av)	0	10
Orange syrup, diluted, 1 cup	66	0	20
Orange juice, 1 cup, 8 ozs.	46	0	26
Papaya, ½ medium, 5 ozs.	58 (av)	0	14
Parsnips, boiled, ½ cup, 2½ ozs.	97	0	15
Pasta			
Capellini, cooked, 1 cup, 6 ozs.	45	1	53
Fettucine, cooked, 1 cup, 6 ozs.	32	1	57
Gnocchi, cooked, 1 cup, 5 ozs.	68	3	71
Linguine thick, cooked, 1 cup, 6 ozs.	46 (av)	1	56
Linguine thin, cooked, 1 cup, 6 ozs.	55 (av)	1	56
Macaroni, cooked, 1 cup, 5 ozs.	45	1	52
Macaroni & Cheese Dinner™, Kraft, packaged, cooked, 1 cup, 7 ozs.	64	17	48
Ravioli, meat-filled, cooked, 1 cup, 9 ozs.	39	8	32
Spaghetti, white, cooked, 1 cup, 6 ozs.	41 (av)	1	52
Spaghetti, whole wheat, cooked, 1 cup, 6 ozs.	37 (av)	1	48
Spirali, durum, cooked, 1 cup, 6 ozs.	43	1	56
Star Pastina, cooked, 1 cup, 6 ozs.	38	1	56
Tortellini, cheese, cooked, 8 ozs.	50	6	26
Vermicelli, cooked, 1 cup, 6 ozs.	35	0	42
Pastry, flaky, ⅛ of double crust, 2 ozs.	59	15	24
Pea soup, split with ham, canned, 1 cup, Wil-Pak Foods, 5½ ozs.	66	7	56
Peach, fresh, 1 medium, 3 ozs.	28	0	7
canned, heavy syrup, ½ cup, 4 ozs.	58	0	26
canned, light syrup, ½ cup, 4 ozs.	52	0	18
canned, natural juice, ½ cup, 4 ozs.	30	0	14
Peanuts, roasted, salted, ½ cup, 2 1/2 ozs.	14 (av)	38	16
Pear, fresh, 1 medium, 5 ozs.	38 (av)	0	21
canned in pear juice, ½ cup, 4 ozs.	44	0	13
Peas, green, fresh, frozen, boiled, ½ cup, 2.7 ozs.	48 (av)	0	11
Peas dried, boiled, ½ cup, 2 ozs.	22	0	7

Food	Glycemic Index	Fat (g per svg.)	CHO (g per svg.)
Pineapple, fresh, 2 slices, 4 ozs.	66	0	10
Pineapple juice, unsweetened, canned, 8 ozs.	46	0	34
Pinto beans, canned, ½ cup, 4 ozs.	45	1	18
Pinto beans, soaked, boiled, ½ cup, 3 ozs.	39	0	22
Pita bread, whole wheat, 6½ inch loaf, 2 ozs.	57	2	35
Pizza, cheese and tomato, 2 slices, 8 ozs.	60	22	56
Plums, 1 medium, 2 ozs.	39 (av)	0	7
Popcorn, light, microwave, 2 cups (popped)	55	3	12
Potatoes			
Desirée, peeled, boiled, 1 medium, 4 ozs.	101	0	13
French fries, large, 4.3 ozs.	75	26	49
instant mashed potatoes, Carnation Foods™, ½ cup, 3½ ozs.	86	2	14
new, unpeeled, boiled, 5 small (cocktail), 6 ozs.	62 (av)	0	23
new, canned, drained, 5 small, 6 ozs.	61	0	23
red-skinned, peeled, boiled, 1 medium, 4 ozs.	88 (av)	0	15
red-skinned, baked in oven (no fat), 1 medium, 4 ozs.	93 (av)	0	15
red-skinned, mashed, ½ cup, 4 ozs.	91 (av)	0	16
red-skinned, microwaved, 1 medium, 4 ozs.	79	0	15
sweet potato, peeled, boiled, ½ cup mashed, 3 ozs.	54 (av)	0	20
white-skinned, peeled, boiled, 1 medium, 4 ozs.	63 (av)	0	24
white-skinned, with skin, baked in oven (no fat), 1 medium, 4 ozs.	85 (av)	0	30
white-skinned, mashed, ½ cup, 4 ozs.	70 (av)	0	20
white-skinned, with skin, microwaved, 1 medium, 4 ozs.	82	0	29
Sebago, peeled, boiled, 1 medium, 4 ozs.	87	0	13
Potato chips, plain, 14 pieces, 1 oz.	54 (av)	11	15
Pound cake, 1 slice, homemade, 3 ozs.	54	15	42
Power Bar™, Performance, Chocolate, 1 bar	58	2	45
Premium saltine crackers, 8 crackers, 1 oz.	74	3	17
Pretzels, 1 oz.	83	1	22
Puffed Wheat™, Quaker, breakfast cereal, 2 cups, 1 oz.	67	0	22
Pumpernickel bread, whole grain, 2 slices	51	2	30
Pumpkin, peeled, boiled, mashed, ½ cup, 4 ozs.	75	0	6
Raisins, ¼ cup, 1 oz.	64	0	28
Raisin Bran™, Kellogg's, breakfast cereal, ¾ cup, 1.3 ozs.	73	0	32
Ravioli, meat-filled, cooked, 1 cup, 9 ozs.	39	8	32
Rice			
Basmati, white, boiled, 1 cup, 7 ozs.	58	0	50

Food	Glycemic Index	Fat (g per svg.)	CHO (g per svg.)
Brown, 1 cup, 6 ozs.	55 (av)	0	37
Converted™, Uncle Ben's, 1 cup, 6 ozs.	44	0	38
Instant, cooked, 1 cup, 6 ozs.	87	0	37
Long grain, white, 1 cup, 6 ozs.	56 (av)	0	42
Parboiled, 1 cup, 6 ozs.	48	0	38
Rice bran, 1 tablespoon	19	2	5
Rice cakes, plain, 3 cakes, 1 oz.	82	1	23
Short grain, white, 1 cup, 6 ozs.	72	0	42
Rice Chex™, General Mills, breakfast cereal, 1¼ cups, 1 oz.	89	0	27
Rice Krispies™, Kellogg's, breakfast cereal, 1¼ cups, 1 oz.	82	0	26
Rice vermicelli, cooked, 6 ozs.	58	0	48
Roll (bread), Kaiser, 1 roll, 2 ozs.	73	2	39
Romano (cranberry) beans, boiled, ½ cup, 3 ozs.	46	0	21
Rutabaga, peeled, boiled, ½ cup, 2.6 ozs.	72	0	3
Rye bread, 1 slice, 1 oz.	65	1	15
Ryvita™ Tasty Dark Rye Whole Grain Crisp Bread, 2 slices, ⅔ oz.	69	1	16
Sausages, smoked link, pork and beef, fried, 2½ ozs.	28	29	5
Semolina, cooked, ⅔ cup, 6 ozs.	55	0	17
Shortbread, 4 small cookies, 1 oz.	64	7	19
Shredded Wheat™, Post, breakfast cereal, 1 oz.	83	1	23
Shredded wheat, 1 biscuit, ⅙ oz.	62	0	19
Skittles Original Fruit Bite Size Candies™, 2.3 oz. pk.	70	3	59
Smacks™, Kellogg's, breakfast cereal, ¾ cup, 1 oz.	56	1	24
Snickers™, 2.2 oz. bar	41	15	36
Social Tea™ biscuits, Nabisco, 4 cookies, ⅔ oz.	55	3	13
Soft drink, Fanta™, 1 can, 12 ozs.	68	0	47
Soups			
Black bean soup, ½ cup, 4½ ozs.	64	2	19
Green pea soup, canned, ready to serve, 1 cup, 9 ozs.	66	3	27
Lentil soup, Unico, canned, 1 cup, 8 ozs.	44	1	24
Pea soup, split, with ham, Wil-Pak Foods, 1 cup, 5½ ozs.	66	7	56
Tomato soup, canned, 1 cup, 9 ozs.	38	4	33
Sourdough bread, 1 slice, 1½ ozs.	52	1	20
Rye bread, Arnold's, 1 slice, 1½ ozs.	57	1	21
Soy beans, boiled, ½ cup, 3 ozs.	18 (av)	7	10
Soy milk, 1 cup, 8 ozs.	31	7	14
Spaghetti, white, cooked, 1 cup	41 (av)	1	52

FOOD	GLYCEMIC INDEX	FAT (G PER SVG.)	CHO (G PER SVG.)
Spaghetti, whole wheat, cooked, 1 cup, 5 ozs.	37 (av)	1	48
Special K™, Kellogg's, breakfast cereal, 1 cup, 1 oz.	66	0	22
Spirali, durum, cooked, 1 cup, 6 ozs.	43	1	56
Split pea soup, 8 ozs.	60	4	38
Split peas, yellow, boiled, ½ cup, 3½ ozs.	32	0	21
Sponge cake plain, 1 slice, 3 ½ ozs.	46	4	32
Sports drinks			
Gatorade™ 1 cup, 8 ozs.	78	0	14
Isostar, 1 cup, 8 ozs.	73	0	18
Sportsplus, 1 cup, 8 ozs.	74	0	17
Sports bars			
Power Bar™, Performance Chocolate Bar, 1 bar	58	2	45
Stoned wheat thins, 3 crackers, ⅔ oz.	67	2	15
Strawberry Nestle Quik™ (made with water), 3 teaspoons	64	0	14
Strawberry jam, 1 tablespoon	51	0	18
Sucrose, 1 teaspoon	65 (av)	0	4
Syrup, fruit flavored, diluted, 1 cup	66	0	20
Sweet corn, canned, drained, ½ cup, 3 ozs.	55 (av)	1	16
Sweet potato, peeled, boiled, ½ cup mashed, 3 ozs.	54 (av)	0	20
Taco shells, 2 shells, 1 oz.	68	5	17
Tapioca pudding, boiled with whole milk, 1 cup, 10 ozs.	81	13	51
Taro, peeled, boiled, ½ cup, 2 ozs.	54	0	23
Team Flakes™, Nabisco, breakfast cereal, ¾ cup, 1 oz.	82	0	25
Tofu frozen dessert, nondairy, low fat, 2 ozs.	115	1	21
Tomato soup, canned, 1 cup, 9 ozs.	38	4	33
Tortellini, cheese, cooked, 8 ozs.	50	6	26
Total™, General Mills, breakfast cereal, ¾ cup, 1 oz.	76	1	24
Twix Chocolate Caramel Cookie™, 2, 2 ozs.	44	14	37
Vanilla wafers, 7 cookies, 1 oz.	77	4	21
Vermicelli, cooked, 1 cup, 6 ozs.	35	0	42
Vitasoy™ Soy milk, creamy original, 1 cup, 8 ozs.	31	7	14
Waffles, plain, frozen, 4 inch square, 1 oz.	76	3	13
Water crackers, 3 king size crackers, ⅔ oz.	78	2	18
Watermelon, 1 cup, 5 ozs.	72	0	8
Weetabix™ breakfast cereal, 2 biscuits, 1.2 ozs.	75	1	28
White bread, 1 slice, 1 oz.	70 (av)	1	12
Whole wheat bread, 1 slice, 1 oz.	69 (av)	1	13

Food	Glycemic Index	Fat (g per svg.)	CHO (g per svg.)
Yam, boiled, 3 ozs.	51	0	31
Yogurt			
nonfat, fruit flavored, with sugar, 8 ozs.	33	0	30
nonfat, plain, artificial sweetener, 8 ozs.	14	0	17
nonfat, fruit flavored, artificial sweetener, 8 ozs.	14	0	16

GLYCEMIC INDEX TESTING

If you are a food manufacturer, you may be interested in having the glycemic index of some of your products tested on a fee-for-service basis. For more information, contact either:

Glycaemic Index Testing Inc.
135 Mavety Street
Toronto, Ontario
Canada M6P 2L8
E mail: thomas.wolever@utoronto.ca

or

Sydney University Glycaemic Index Research
Service (SUGIRS)
Department of Biochemistry
University of Sydney
NSW 2006 Australia
Fax: (61) (2) 9351-6022
E-mail: j.brandmiller@staff.usyd.edu.au

FOR MORE INFORMATION

REGISTERED DIETITIANS

Registered Dietitians (R.D.s) are nutrition experts who provide nutritional assessment and guidance and support with weight loss. Check for the initials "R.D." after the name to identify qualified dietitians who provide the highest standard of care to their clients. Glycemic index is part of their training so all dietitians should be able to help in applying the principles in this guide, but some dietitians do specialize in certain areas. If you want more detailed advice on losing weight and the glycemic index just ask the dietitian whether this is a specialty when you make your appointment.

Dietitians work in hospitals and often run their own private practices as well. For a list of dietitians in your area, contact the American Dietetic Association (ADA) Consumer Nutrition Hotline (1-800-366-1655) or visit ADA's home page at the address below. You can also check the Yellow Pages under "Dietitians."

The American Dietetic Association
216 West Jackson Boulevard
Chicago, IL 60606
Phone: 1-800-877-1600
Fax: 1-312-899-1979
Web site: http://www.eatright.org/

PRIMARY CARE PHYSICIANS

If you think you need help with a weight problem, it's always a good idea to see your primary care physician for an evaluation.

COMMUNITY SUPPORT GROUPS

Many communities offer support groups targeting people who are trying to lose weight. Your primary care physician or local hospital may be able to direct you to a support group best suited to your needs.

WEIGHT LOSS ORGANIZATIONS

To find a weight-loss organization in your area, check the Yellow Pages under "Weight Control Services." Be aware, however, that not all weight-loss organizations are reputable. Check with your physician to make sure the group you'd like to join can help you lose weight safely.

DIABETES ORGANIZATIONS

Extra weight can make diabetes (and its complications) worse. For more information about living with and controlling your diabetes, contact the following:

The American Diabetes Association
1660 Duke Street
Alexandria, VA 22314
Phone: 1-800-ADA-DISC (1-800-232-3472)
Web site: http://www.diabetes.org/

Canadian Diabetes Association
National Office
15 Toronto St. Ste. #800
Toronto, ON M5C 2E3
Phone: 1-416-363-3373
1-800-BANTING (1-800-226-8464)
Web site: http://www.diabetes.ca/

NATURAL OVENS ORDERING INFORMATION

Natural Ovens of Manitowoc
4300 County Trunk CR
P.O. Box 730
Manitowoc WI 54221-073
Telephone: 1-800-772-0730
Fax: 920-758-2594
http://www.naturalovens.com/

ACKNOWLEDGMENTS

We would like to acknowledge the extraordinary efforts of Johanna Burani and Linda Rao, who adapted this book—and the other books in *The Glucose Revolution Pocket Guide* series—for North American readers. Together they have worked to ensure that every piece of information is accurate and appropriate for readers in the U.S. and Canada.

ABOUT THE AUTHORS

Kaye Foster-Powell, B.Sc., M. Nutr. & Diet., is an accredited dietitian-nutritionist in both public and private practice in New South Wales, Australia. A graduate of the University of Sydney (B.Sc., 1987; Masters of Nutrition and Dietetics, 1994), she has extensive experience in diabetes management and has researched practical applications of the glycemic index over the last five years. A co-author of *The Glucose Revolution* and all the titles in *The Glucose Revolution Pocket Guide* Series, she lives in Sydney, Australia.

Jennie Brand-Miller, Ph.D., Associate Professor of Human Nutrition in the Human Nutrition Unit, Department of Biochemistry, University of Sydney, Australia, is widely recognized as one of the world's leading authorities on the glycemic index. She received her B.Sc. (1975) and Ph.D. (1979) degrees from the Department of Food Science and Technology at the University of New South Wales, Australia. She is the editor of the *Proceedings of the Nutrition Society of Australia* and a member of the Scientific Consultative Committee of the Australian Nutrition Foundation. She has written more than 200 research papers, including 60 on the glycemic index of foods. A co-author of *The Glucose Revolution* and all the titles in *The Glucose*

Revolution Pocket Guide Series, she lives in Sydney, Australia.

Thomas M.S. Wolever, M.D., Ph.D., another of the world's leading researchers of the glycemic index, is Professor in the Department of Nutritional Sciences, University of Toronto, and a member of the Division of Endocrinology and Metabolism, St. Michael's Hospital, Toronto. He is a graduate of Oxford University (B.A., M.A., M.B., B.Ch., M.Sc., and D.M.). He received his Ph.D. at the University of Toronto. His research since 1980 has focused on the glycemic index of foods and the prevention of type 2 diabetes. A co-author of *The Glucose Revolution* and all the titles in *The Glucose Revolution Pocket Guide* Series, he lives in Toronto, Canada.

Stephen Colagiuri, M.D., is the President of the Australian Diabetes Society, director of the Diabetes Center, and head of the Department of Endocrinology, Metabolism, and Diabetes at the Prince of Wales Hospital, Randwick, New South Wales, Australia. He is a graduate of the University of Sydney (M.B.B.S., 1970) and a member of the Royal Australasian College of Physicians (1977). He has joint academic appointments at the University of New South Wales. He has authored more than 100 scientific papers, many concerned with the importance of carbohydrate in the diet of people with diabetes. A co-author of *The Glucose Revolution* and several other titles in *The Glucose Revolution Pocket Guide* Series, he lives in Sydney, Australia.

Johanna Burani, M.S., R.D., C.D.E., is a registered dietitian and certified diabetes educator with more than 10 years experience in nutritional counseling. She specializes in designing individual meal plans based on low glycemic-index food choices. The adapter of *The Glucose Revolution* and co-adapter, with Linda Rao, of all the titles in *The Glucose Revolution Pocket Guide* Series, she is the author of seven books and professional manuals, and lives in Mendham, New Jersey.

Linda Rao, M.Ed., a freelance writer and editor, has been writing and researching health topics for the past 11 years. Her work has appeared in several national publications, including *Prevention* and *USA Today*. She serves as a contributing editor for *Prevention* Magazine and is the co-adapter, with Johanna Burani, of all the titles in *The Glucose Revolution Pocket Guide* Series. She lives in Allentown, Pennsylvania.

The Glucose Revolution begins here . . .

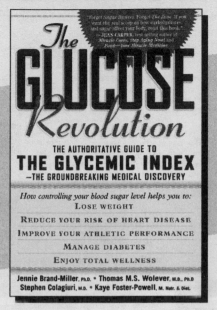

THE GLUCOSE REVOLUTION
The Authoritative Guide to the Glycemic Index—
The Groundbreaking Medical Discovery

National Bestseller!

"Forget *Sugar Busters*. Forget *The Zone*. If you want the real scoop on how carbohydrates and sugar affect your body, read this book by the world's leading researchers on the subject. It's the authoritative, last word on choosing foods to control your blood sugar."

—Jean Carper, best-selling author of *Miracle Brain, Miracle Cures, Stop Aging Now!* and *Food—Your Miracle Medicine*

ISBN 1-56924-660-2 • $14.95

. . . and continues with these other
Glucose Revolution Pocket Guides

The Glucose Revolution Pocket Guide to
THE TOP 100 LOW GLYCEMIC FOODS

The best of the best in low glycemic index foods
The slow digestion and gradual rise and fall in blood sugar levels after a food with a low glycemic index has benefits for many people. Today we know the glycemic index of hundreds of different generic and name-brand foods, which have been tested following a standardized method. Now *The Top 100 Low Glycemic Foods* makes it easy to enjoy those slowly digested carbohydrates every day for better blood sugar control, weight loss, a healthy heart, and peak athletic performance.
ISBN 1-56924-678-5 • $4.95

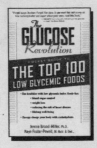

The Glucose Revolution Pocket Guide to
DIABETES

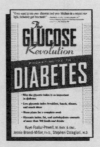

Help control your diabetes with low glycemic index foods
This basic guide to the glycemic index and diabetes allows people with type 1 and type 2 diabetes to make more informed choices about their diets. Topics covered include why many traditionally "taboo" foods don't cause the unfavorable effects on blood sugar levels they were believed to have, and why diets based on low G.I. foods improve blood sugar control. Also covered are how to include more of the right kinds of carbohydrates in your diet, the optimum diet for people with diabetes, practical hints for meal preparation and tips to help make the glycemic index work throughout the day, a week of low G.I. menus, G.I. success stories, and more.
ISBN 1-56924-675-0 • $4.95

The Glucose Revolution Pocket Guide to
SPORTS NUTRITION

Eat to compete better than ever before
Serious athletes and weekend warriors can gain a winning edge by manipulating the glycemic index of their diets. Now this at-a-glance guide shows how to use the glycemic index to boost athletic performance, enhance stamina, and prevent fatigue. Subjects covered include energy charging with carbohydrates, eating for competing, refueling hints, menu plans and case studies, and the glycemic index, fat and carbohydrate content of more than 300 foods and drinks.
ISBN 1-56924-676-9 • $4.95

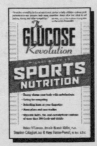